Pharmaceutical Energetics

by the same author

The Spirit of the Blood
Interpreting Laboratory Tests Through the Lens of Chinese Medicine
Randine Lewis
ISBN 978 1 83997 053 5
eISBN 978 1 83997 054 2

Birthing the Tao
Supporting the Incarnating Soul's Development through Pregnancy or Rebirthing
Randine Lewis
Foreword by Lorie Dechar
ISBN 978 1 78775 999 2
eISBN 978 1 83997 003 0

of related interest

Kigo
Exploring the Spiritual Essence of Acupuncture Points Through the Changing Seasons
Lorie Eve Dechar
Foreword by Randine Lewis
ISBN 978 1 78775 256 6
eISBN 978 1 78775 257 3

Applying Stems and Branches Acupuncture in Clinical Practice
Dynamic Dualities in Classical Chinese Medicine
Joan Duveen
Foreword by Tae Hunn Lee
ISBN 978 1 78775 370 9
eISBN 978 1 78775 371 6

PHARMACEUTICAL ENERGETICS

Analyzing Common Drugs Through
the Lens of Chinese Medicine

RANDINE LEWIS

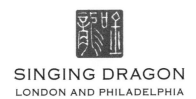

SINGING DRAGON
LONDON AND PHILADELPHIA

First published in Great Britain in 2025 by Singing Dragon,
an imprint of Jessica Kingsley Publishers
Part of John Murray Press

2

A CIP catalogue record for this title is available from the
British Library and the Library of Congress

ISBN 978 1 80501 031 9
eISBN 978 1 80501 032 6

Printed and bound in the United States by Integrated Books International

Jessica Kingsley Publishers' policy is to use papers that are natural, renewable
and recyclable products and made from wood grown in sustainable
forests. The logging and manufacturing processes are expected to conform
to the environmental regulations of the country of origin.

Singing Dragon
Carmelite House
50 Victoria Embankment
London EC4Y 0DZ

www.singingdragon.com

John Murray Press
Part of Hodder & Stoughton Limited
An Hachette UK Company

Contents

Acknowledgements

No work in this field can be a solitary endeavor. The *Su Wen* stresses the importance of taking the wisdom of antiquity and making it relevant to the present. I continue to be influenced by those who remain steeped in the infinite intelligence and eternal guidance the Tao provides, and are willing to share it where it is most relevant today. Nowhere has this been more evident than gathering with treasured colleagues Lorie Dechar, Heiner Fruehauf, Alexander Love, Brandt Stickley, and Will Morris, for our Integral Chinese Medicine Collective, where our shared presence intensifies the potential this wisdom tradition is capable of, beaming forth in delight of the unified field.

I'd like to convey my deepest gratitude for those whose lives are devoted to embodying the wisdom tradition of the Tao, especially my primary teacher, Jeffrey Yuen, without whom none of this knowledge would have come forth. Additionally, some of Master Yuen's generous senior students like Cissy Majabe and Mona Dinari have contributed their notes and expertise when mine felt lacking. And to the next generation of brilliant practitioners like my son-in-law, Browning Smith, who is always eager to speak Chinese medicine, and my daughter, Theresa Johnson, may you take this work to the next level, and continue to make junction with its ever-present emergence.

Introduction

Until we become the medicine,
We will not overcome what sickens us.

When I began studying Eastern medicine, I had already been steeped in the Western reductionist mindset where the science of matter rules. When I enrolled in Chinese medical school, eager to learn the ancient secrets of the art of healing, I was amazed at the vast chasms between these two thought systems. In one, matter ruled; the other one placed primary emphasis on the Heart Mind, which energy then followed, determining how matter behaved. I was challenged to leave behind all I knew about Western medicine and enter into a different thought system altogether. In spite of some of the issues I had with Western medicine, my mind still railed. I thought I'd be adding knowledge, not subtracting. Because I knew Western medicine first, I had to try to fit Chinese medicine into my Western understanding. The disadvantage was it didn't work very well. The advantage was that it gave me a front-row seat to all of my biases and ways of thinking that were not in alignment with the Way and its power. Over the next few decades I continued challenging my Western mindset and very slowly opened up to a different way of approaching both, where Eastern philosophy became my prevailing mindset, to which Western concepts could be applied or discarded. The Taoist philosophy behind classical Chinese medicine has to be lived, not just studied. It is truly a lifelong practice of attempting to be rooted in the Tao, until eventually we become steeped in its Way.

Years ago, I was invited to teach at a doctoral program of Asian medicine with an emphasis on spiritual cultivation and understanding the Taoist classics. One of the integrative doctoral classes I co-teach is entitled *Pharmaceutical Energetics*. Along with its partner, *Laboratory Analysis*, it raises the academic standards for Chinese medical understanding. These classes present the prevailing medical approach of analyzing blood work and prescribing pharmaceuticals not as a stand-alone system to be honored, respected, and figuratively bowed to, but instead to be critiqued and put under the scrutiny of East Asian medical energetics. These disciplines are in their infancy, as very little is written with regard to how to keep the Chinese medical lens front and center. I was asked to write *The Spirit of the Blood* (Lewis, 2022) first, and thought that would be the end of it. But as often happens, the Tao has other plans.

Not too long ago, I was staying at a friend's house and she had her television on in the background most of the day. After not watching mainstream TV for decades, it was unnerving to hear advertisements for prescription medications every few minutes. In one, Jennifer Aniston was having difficulty sleeping, and her phone's little sheep counting sleep app was humorously giving her a hard time for outlasting it. It was cute, funny, and catchy; and like most of the other ads, it ended up with "Ask your doctor…" for whatever medication was being peddled. It was quite shocking to me, and seemed ethically questionable, kind of like cigarette commercials in the 1960s trying to convince consumers that it was cool to smoke. I felt as if I was plunged into another reality where people weren't even questioning what their minds were being fed. I don't think it's funny or cool to be asking your doctor for prescription sleep meds that you happen to see on a TV commercial. But those who practice Chinese medicine don't tend to think like the general pharmaceutical consuming public. We question the prevailing narrative, which makes very little sense, even to some of its most avid consumers. We are rarely impressed by double-blinded-placebo-controlled-repeatable-studies, most of which are paid for by pharmaceutical companies. We'd rather read a discourse between the Yellow Emperor and Qi Bo on the nature of healing than try to squeeze our vast healing tradition into something called "evidence based," which doesn't come close to validating the true nature of healing. Yet instead of discarding the evidence-based approach, we'll use it to understand the patterns behind disease and why medication is rarely the long-term solution. No matter how we look at the process of healing, however, it always seems to end up back in the same place—East Asian medicine and the wisdom philosophy on which it is based simply makes the most sense. Once again, the sun is setting on the West and is rising in the East. I guess it's time to write another book.

Like many others in this healing tradition, I'm intrigued by life's myriad transformations, of how we come into being, and the mystery of our own passing. We come from and return to the great unknown. In between, we can be assured of one thing: we will die. Much, if not most, of the modern Western pharmacopeia is an attempt to avoid the one unavoidable thing. And we go to war against its allies, taking antivirals, antibiotics, and anti-hypertensives. We battle natural substances like cholesterol, mask the messages pain can convey, and pretend we are living a healthy life. We take drugs for the side effects that other drugs cause. Even the process of death is usually narcotized so we don't get to experience what it's like to journey beyond this plane of existence. The Dalai Lama is quoted as saying, "Man lives as if he is never going to die, and then dies having never really lived." Once we have accepted the fact of our inevitable death and stop fighting it, we can let go of some of the untruths we've unconsciously accepted and begin to truly live as nature intended, to find harmony within our internal and external environments. We were meant to live this exciting, unpredictable, sometimes dangerous, sometimes threatening life, with all of its unforeseeable vicissitudes.

Dying, which is part of it, is not to be feared nor avoided; in fact, it may be the greatest adventure, and the very reason we were given life. Chapter 7 of the *Huainanzi* speculates that perhaps desiring life and practicing the healing traditions is a delusion, and death might be the ultimate blessing—a respite from all this toil. The Taoists, like many other ancient traditions, practiced *dying every day*, and as they released attachments that held them down along the way, their bodies often lived well past a hundred years. United with the source, they knew when their earthly time was up, and let their bodies fall away as their true being returned to its cosmic home. We all have this knowing deep inside; it seems we were born with a premonitory longing and hopeful recognition that there is something eternal within us that actually does go on forever. Some call it the soul; others refer to the indwelling spirit, Atman, or higher self. If we know the Yang yet keep to the Yin, as the *Tao te Ching* instructs us, perhaps we'll find it.

The meaning of life, according to ancient Eastern philosophical views, is to discover our destiny, whose purpose is to then live out the expression of our true nature, at one with Heaven and Earth. Our souls are encapsulations of the One celestial spirit, Big Shen, that condenses to live as a specific spectrum of energy spanning time, space, and dimensionality. This view is not limited to enlightened sages from the East, however. Niels Bohr said that everything we call real is made of things that cannot be regarded as real. Quantum science posits that DNA itself, the foundation of our supposed finite physical selves, is actually a liquid crystalline substance that receives energetic information from the environment through the biofield in the form of imagery and archetypes which are then translated into three-dimensional holographic images. From the energy field where protons meet black holes, Ling Zi 靈 子 (literally soul children) are described as the most minute spiritual particles, which the brain receives, organizes, and interprets into a seeming solid reality, which is actually orchestrated by a force higher than our supposed finite selves.

Our seven senses (hearing, seeing, smelling, tasting, touching, thinking, and feeling) have been conditioned to create projections based on learned societal agreements. The "input" our senses convey is received by an energetic contraction that produces a sense of a separate identity, along with its interpretations and beliefs. And we protect this contraction as if our lives depend on it. But only the illusory identity of the ego dies. We actually become quite disturbed if our imagined reality breaks down. We develop states of disease, aches, and pains; our five Zang become disturbed, and the Qi may run counterflow. And we run to our doctors to be told what's wrong and how they can remedy it for us.

If we remain present to our supposed "difficulties," our consciousness can view these challenges as invitations to see that our projected world is an illusion, and we are not actually limited to space and time. While this may fly in the face of conventional medical dogma, ancient Taoist wisdom viewed our animate bodies as ensouled functions that interface with other planes of existence. Our meridians, which could be seen as networks of vibration, coexist in the multiverse, beyond space and time, and while they materialize into this three-dimensional bodily form, they are not limited by it. That is, unless we believe that they are.

While the corporeal soul and its distortions thankfully come to an end, the eternal energy of the ethereal soul does not. In the ancient Aramaic language, the word death is understood to mean "existing elsewhere." When the microcosmic body comes to an end, *elsewhere* becomes the wondrous mystery of the macrocosm. During earthly life, existing elsewhere means we are trapped in one of the egoic powers of the seven Po, which live either in the past or the future, taking us out of present time access to pure Shen. Once we learn to see through the distortions of the ego and come to know the eternal nature of our authentic selves all the way down to our marrow, what could we possibly have to fear? We are given a different directive to follow, based not on symptom resolution or avoidance of the body's death, but on transcending our limitations and expanding ever beyond the borders of our supposed finitude. It is a joyful thing to see through our own hauntings, both personally and collectively, and come to know ourselves as the Tao. We have the entire universe behind us, if we will tune into its ever-beckoning call.

The *Nei Jing Su Wen* tells us in Chapter 26 that *the Heart is the rooting of life* and in Chapter 8 that *All diseases are rooted in spirit*. When we ail it is because we have lost harmony with the Heart, the home of the spirit and the origin of all true healing. If we don't discover our true nature and the very purpose of our souls, we will always feel that something is a bit off, like a low-grade discontent. And we will want to get away from this feeling, although it is meant to propel us into awakening, not to find ways to deaden our discomfort.

Our vastness is incomprehensible to the standardized ways we've been taught to perceive life, health, and medicine. We are mesmerized by the scientific method under which we've been indoctrinated, and our belief in its reductionist paradigm swears allegiance to the mechanics of matter as the highest truth. Most patients with whom I have worked throughout the years don't respect the medical system they've been pretty much forced to use; they don't want to be squeezed into its diagnostic parameters and don't want to take the medications they've been prescribed. Deep inside they know that there is a miraculous healing power within; they just haven't been shown how to tap into this energy potential that lives within their own Heart. Their reliance on doctors and external medical systems, which is usually all they've ever known, actually prevents them from accessing this power. The Blood (matter) follows the Qi, which follows the Heart-Mind. When they discover another way to approach their healing, however, the predominant Western medical model makes very little sense. Why? Because we have the whole equation backward; the Heart-Mind is not meant to follow the Blood, and we know it.

When I first began practicing, East Asian medicine was rarely anyone's first choice. Only after Western medicine had failed them, and they had nowhere else to turn, would they try acupuncture and herbs. Decades later, the conventional medical system is less personal, more automated, and frankly far more confusing. For issues like trauma, limb replacements, and life-saving intervention, Western medicine shines. Disciplines like bio-field healing provide exciting potentials for the future of scientific medical advancement. But for healing, or even health management, it is an outdated system that just doesn't work, and more people are looking for alternatives.

This is not an anti-conventional medicine book. Since conventional medicine rarely focuses on the origin of disease, I will be coming from what might be considered a radical approach of trying to reach the root of healing. Like the function of my practice and teaching, the goal of this work is to understand the energies behind the development of disease processes, so we may heal the body, mind, and life and avoid unnecessary medications. Many, if not most, chronic disease processes are simply the result of living out of balance.

Nor is this book an encyclopedia of nutritional supplements that you can take for certain ailments. There are many amazing books and naturopathic and functional medical physicians who can guide you toward specific natural remedies. Certainly, topical aloe vera might be preferable to hydrocortisone cream if it can get the job done. But is taking handfuls of nutraceuticals or bio-identicals all that different from taking a synthesized chemical? Neither reach the root. My aim is to provide another way of viewing the energetics of the body altogether, according to the principles of nature, like the Chinese physicians of antiquity did. When there is pain, the Qi is not flowing. Instead of masking the pain—a form of resistance—attend to it. Go right into the center of it with curiosity and see what it has to teach you. What is obstructing the smooth flow of Qi? Could it be the thousands of times you said yes when you really meant no?

I used to get migraine headaches that started in my twenties. While they weren't a daily occurrence, when I got one, it was debilitating. Always preceded by an aura, an hour later I would be in bed in a darkened room, usually in tears as the pain gripped my brain. I initially consulted a doctor and was prescribed a triptan and ibuprofen, which didn't work very well, but as they sat in my purse they gave me a sense of security that at least I had something to take should an aura come on. Years later, acupuncture and herbs were much more effective at resolving the pain, but didn't keep the headaches from recurring. As I became more conscious of the relationship between my outer and inner world, I started to notice the headaches would often come on after periods of stress had passed.

One day, toward the end of a busy retreat I was conducting at a resort outside Austin, my vision started to go askew. I had just been teaching the participants about how to learn from their pain. As the blind spot in my visual field intensified and I anticipated the inevitable pounding head pain, I turned the attendees over to a co-facilitator while I asked one of our acupuncturists to give me a treatment. After he got a few needles in, my body almost revolted. *No more!* I was simply no longer going to be at the mercy of these headaches. I asked him to remove the needles. Alone in my room, instead of pleading for the pain to stop, I became curious about what it really meant. Sure, I knew about the vascular changes that caused migraines, but that was a surface understanding. I wanted to know the deeper cause. What was behind these recurrent symptoms? Not the physiologic explanation, but what was this process actually there to reveal to me? Nothing happens in the Tao by accident, and I was finally ready to experience the answer. As my attention went right into the center of the pain behind my eye, I became aware of a circle of throbbing red heat about six feet in diameter extending out from the right side of my head where the pain began, at the Gallbladder meridian. And it was mad, red hot mad. As I stayed with the sensation, I became aware of the times in my recent past when I made decisions based on fear of hurting other people's feelings, which placed me in a position of feeling victimized and resentful. I got the message that this behavior had to stop, at which time a wave of compassion for my misunderstanding moved through me and the headache stopped, just like that. I haven't had another migraine since. While I still might default to people-pleasing behavior, it is now conscious. The headache did its job. It was never there to punish, but to reveal.

This book is not going to be about what to do when you get a headache either, but this example does bring up an important point. We are a pain-avoiding society. Admittedly, it is hard to function optimally when we hurt, and pain may mean something's wrong. But it may also mean something needs to be attended to and changed. When my objective was to stop the pain, even with acupuncture, I couldn't learn from it. Symptoms do not mean failure; they indicate there is a conflict. The body speaks its own unique language, and when we tune our listening inward to heed its messages, the unconscious becomes conscious, and we are on our way toward a cure. When we take analgesics to cover over our discomfort, on the other hand, it produces a state of Cold in the Liver. Energetically this means that we are resisting the experience of pain that is inviting us to change. A healthy Liver keeps our Qi flowing smoothly, and also invites transformation. When we are in a state of resistance, the Liver energies become stagnant, and we can't change. Stagnant Liver energies cannot metabolize medicines like analgesics very well, either, producing a vicious cycle of insidious iatrogenic symptoms within a web from which we can't seem to escape.

Sometimes medications actually obstruct our ability to truly heal. Popping a pill is less troubling than learning to say no when it might hurt someone's feelings. Taking a drug to control blood sugar might be easier than recognizing why we comfort ourselves with chocolate cake. And taking antidepressants might be less complicated than leaving a toxic marriage. While it might feel daunting to take the responsibility for our health out of the hands of our physicians and into our own, it is also supremely empowering. Behind every issue is what the Classics describe as the *trigger that set it in motion*; in other words, the root of the imbalance. When it is identified, the cure is at hand and we don't need to become overly concerned with the state of the branch symptoms.

We who practice this medicine would be wise to ask ourselves, as I was asked many years ago by my teacher Jeffrey Yuen, "What system are you loyal to?" Do you utilize the tools of conventional biomedicine first, and resort to Chinese medicine when all else fails? Are you on medication because Chinese medicine isn't powerful enough to address your particular manifestation? Do you pay attention to labs and meds more than tongue and pulse? Where do you place the power of healing? In the hands of the doctors, your own hands, or in the spirit of healing that resides in the Heart of every cell?

Darlene sought help with East Asian medicine when she was 50 years old and her hormones were in a state of flux. She had been experiencing extreme fatigue, anxiety, sleeplessness, and chest pain that would sometimes last up to two days. She previously had a history of low blood pressure and anemia. She did not want to go on medication, which was being strongly encouraged by her physician. Instead, she was taking a grocery bag full of expensive supplements prescribed by a naturopath, which she said didn't make any difference to her symptoms. Her present blood work revealed elevated red and white blood cell counts (with increased eosinophils), increased hemoglobin, elevated thyroid stimulating hormone, hypercholesterolemia, and electrolyte imbalances (anion gap). This particular scenario revealed that she was manifesting an increased level of protection, based on a history of past neglect and trauma. It is not unusual to manifest these types of abnormalities during the perimenopausal years. During this potent time of transformation, the body-mind is given an enormous opportunity (should one accept the invitation) to deal with unresolved issues of the past. Based on analysis of her lab results, tongue, and pulse, and after questioning her about her health, I asked her a single pointed question about her childhood. It was something as simple as: "Who was there to care for you?" As she received the inquiry, her tearful acknowledgement told me we had just found the root, the trigger which set the myriad manifestations of her disturbed internal environment in motion. While she was given acupuncture and herbs to support her, the real work, that of her own Heart, was to recognize all of the ways that she felt she had to protect herself her entire life, and to acknowledge how alone she had always felt. Her Blood was given the opportunity it needed to settle down. She was enormously relieved, and ended up needing no medication (or expensive supplements). She changed from the inside out.

In this work, we will evaluate the most common disease states for which medications are prescribed. We will view the normal physiology of each system; and through the lens of Chinese medicine, how pathophysiology and resultant patterns of imbalance tend to manifest. We will then evaluate the most commonly prescribed pharmaceuticals, and discover how they impact the underlying energetics of the system. Sometimes it is smarter and more compassionate to remain on certain necessary medications. Insulin, for example, is crucial to manage Type 1 diabetes. But more often than not, when we understand the underlying energies, a cure can be obtained without resorting to pharmaceutical remedies. Pharmaceutically altered disease states tend to allow and even reinforce the underlying patterns of imbalance, while their symptoms alone are reduced.

When we can understand what's going on energetically, and apply the therapeutic principles of East Asian medicine, we can work with, rather than against, the medicated disease. Changes in lifestyle, diet, and outlook, and using acupuncture and herbs, can allow most people to taper off most medications. Some are able to go off all of their medications; some remain on one or two. The key here is to understand the energetics of the medicine and allow the individual to regain control over their own health care.

If the purpose of life is to seek pleasure and avoid pain, then that which provides temporary comfort will be highly valued. This type of life is one that tends to remain stuck in patterns of imbalance that manifest illness. Sometimes the best we can do is medicate our discomfort. If, however, the function of life is to learn, grow, transcend limitations, and come to the awareness of our divine nature, then strap in. Life will be exciting and unpredictable. We will be unsettled at times. But if we remain true to ourselves without medicating our discomfort, we will find the answers we have been looking for within. For every lesson learned and imbalance overcome, we will vibrate at a higher state where the previous disease no longer exists.

After years of teaching Chinese medicine, it has been my experience that practitioners in our field usually do not know enough about the energetics of pharmaceuticals to make sense of how they fit into the pattern of the individuals they are treating. Instead, they either ignore the medication, or bow to it, accepting as a fact that their allopathic physician knows more about the patient's health than they or we do. This is simply untrue. *Pharmaceutical*

Energetics will attempt to correct this misperception. We will evaluate each class of drugs, based on their popularity, and provide the energetics of each class through the lens of Chinese medicine; starting with those that impact the Wei Qi, the Blood and Shen, Ying Qi, and Jing:

- Antimicrobials—antibiotics, antivirals, antiparasitics, antifungals
- Antidepressants, anxiolytics, and amphetamines
- Pain relievers, non-steroidal anti-inflammatory drugs (NSAIDs), muscle relaxers, and opioids
- Antihypertensives
- Diabetes, metabolic syndrome, and pharmaceuticals to address both
- Cholesterol-lowering and cardiovascular drugs
- Thyroid and reproductive hormones
- Cancer and chemotherapy

The method we will utilize will be to discover the unique mode of action of each drug: what it is and how it impacts our physiology; what types of Chinese medical patterns contribute to the disease process for which the drug is prescribed; the types of signs and symptoms it aims to alleviate and the mechanism for relief. We'll also explore what the common side effects are and how the drug's actions would be categorized according to East Asian medicinal principles. Then we can ascertain if Chinese medicine can treat the disease process and alleviate the need for the medicine altogether, enhance the actions of the medication, or mitigate its side effects.

It will not be plausible to cover every category of pharmaceutical, but as you work with this process and learn how to evaluate the most common drugs on the market, you should be able to apply this process to other pharmaceuticals as well.

Because the dominant Western mindset is one of allopathic and pharmaceutical reliance, some of the ideas presented may sound extremist or farfetched. Can we expect someone diagnosed with clinical depression to be free of their antidepressants? Can we help someone diagnosed with diabetes or hypercholesteremia give up their meds? What about a cancer diagnosis? Dare we address it with Chinese herbs and acupuncture? We face these dilemmas daily in our practice. While this book may present a radical view to some, it is meant to counter the prevailing medical paradigm. In practice, however, we must take each case individually. Some want to be medication free, and have the inner resources to accomplish this task. Others may not fare so well. This is where medical discernment becomes our greatest asset.

CHAPTER 1

Health Care vs Disease Management

All diseases are rooted in spirit.

—*Ling Shu*, Chapter 8

The eighth chapter of the *Ling Shu* (Spiritual Pivot) begins with a discourse between the mythic emperor Huang Di, who was born through a *surge of the spirits*, and his trusted sage, Qi Bo. Huang Di, one of the best question-askers in history, begins with an offering, where he asserts that the laws of acupuncture must first be rooted in spirit. He then goes on to note that when we don't follow nature's way, the viscera and their substances may become agitated and separate, our spirits become disordered, and we ail. He asks Qi Bo why this is and who's to blame. Is it due to the universal laws of Heaven or does the fault lie with humans who go against nature? Huang Di really knows how to offer up a conundrum, which takes years of cultivation to unpack. Qi Bo presents an equally sagacious reply that Heaven endows the power of virtue 德 when one's head is aligned with one's heart over one's feet, and Earth abides within as Qi. When these two flow harmoniously, there is life. The conversation goes on to describe Essences and Spirits, functions of the Heart-Mind, and how emotional disturbances can injure the Qi, scatter the Spirits, and result in the loss of self.

That, it seems, is the primary cause of disease. We have lost touch with the true unitive self, the conduit where spirits and energy flow between Heaven, which comes first, and Earth, which comes second, according to the *Ling Shu*. While Huang Di and Qi Bo lived during a geocentric period, we have moved through a heliocentric view, and finally to one that recognizes that the celestial laws of Heaven permeate Earth, and it is through the function of being human this order of reality comes to be known and integrated in the human being. Qi Bo asserts that the utmost treatment principle lies with oneness. Note that in order for acupuncture to be successful, we must *move the patient's spirits*. Back in the day, this might have been understood as divining ghostly presences, but today we understand that we must be able to shift the patient's state of consciousness to a vibratory level where healing can take place. There is no real and lasting healing without a corresponding change of Mind. And when we are transformed to this extent, our entire ancestral line changes with us.

While our bodies are made of the fleshy substance of earth, Heaven imparts the gift of conscious animation, providing the enlivening spirits that reside in the human Heart. Our conscious experience of life is almost infinite in potential, limited only by how our conditioned beliefs define us and our earthly expression. These limitations obstruct the flow of Qi and Blood, but thankfully the Xin, Heart-Mind, has the ability to overcome these blockages and ultimately determine our ability to heal.

We live as a much larger spectrum of energy that manifests as a living, breathing, perceiving bodily being, *shenti* 身体, which is not separate from the mental and emotional fluctuations caused by societal, cultural, and environmental factors in this three-dimensional world, and the goal of health is to achieve a balanced state between Heaven and Earth. When we lose harmony with nature, or the Way, we experience states of distress and dis-ease. Our Qi might become depressed. We may contract in fear. We may develop heart palpitations. Every symptom, every discomfort, is therefore an invitation to correct our walk and return to a state of harmonious oneness where the Heart and Spirit return to their rightful place and we will not ail. And lest you think this is only a task that the Taoist immortals undertook, let me quote another well-known healer, who only sounds like a Taoist:

> This is why you become sick and die, for you love what deceives you... Matter
> gives birth to a passion that has no likeness because it proceeds from what is

contrary to nature. Then there arises a disturbance in the whole body... and finally... You shall become satisfied and not be persuaded. You shall be joined in the presence of the likeness of nature.

—*Jesus of Nazareth, Gospel of Mary, 3: 7–12*

And just like our Taoist forebears, we see that it is when we go contrary to nature that we develop disturbances in the body. So, like Huang Di, we might ask where the error lies. Is it with Heaven, nature, society, or humanity itself? And like Qi Bo, we might wax philosophical and answer something like: *Man is not separate from his environment. He has learned to love that which deceives him. He's chosen the easier, softer life of pleasure and comfort, and he has lost his power. He's afraid of discomfort and goes to doctors who prescribe pills to silence the voices of truth within.* Entropy and inertia win. The spirits scatter, the sick get sicker, and the drug companies get richer.

Such is the state of our modern medical industry, which does not empower us to stay well. Very few allopathic physicians speak the language of wellness. How many people do you know who look forward to their annual medical screening because it will substantiate how well they are doing? How many return from their doctor's visits with an open Heart, a new aha, and a plan to live better? Almost everyone, especially those who have been sick in the past, resists slipping on the blood pressure cuff, stepping on the scale, getting needles poked in their veins, and waiting for the dreaded results of how they are actually doing, according to the numbers, and what medication might now be needed to keep them from getting sicker.

A patient who had been diagnosed with and treated for cancer decades ago still dutifully reports back to the cancer seeking team each year, as he was told anyone with cancer has a 70 percent chance of another recurrence. The month his annual comes due, his stress levels go through the roof. *What will they find? Is it back?* I've noticed his otherwise healthy living practices go out the window as he makes himself more prone to becoming sick. When we are in states of distress, we tend to drink more, eat more of the wrong types of food, and exercise and sleep less. When our relationship with our health is based on fear of getting sick, it is not health care at all; for we know that fear and stress lower our immunity and make us prone to a plethora of illness.

While this is obviously not wellness, it is because science and conventional medicine have been in service so long we have become blind to it. When politicians were touting their "I believe in science!" slogans across television screens, some of us with more metaphysical bents were raising eyebrows, quietly thinking, *Hmm... I believe in the nature of the Tao, which modern quantum science is only beginning to touch.*

Even genetic testing, the creme de la creme of modern medicine, does not take the fascinating science of epigenetics into account, the study of how and why certain genes turn on and off in response to environmental cues, emotional reactions, and shifts in our belief patterns. There are even pharmacogenetic tests available that look for genetic variants that impact how one metabolizes and responds to certain pharmaceuticals, steering them toward which medications they should be prescribed. Our DNA is not the source but the conveyance through which the intelligence of life is transmitted. If we lock it in as the primary determinant of our health, the wave of possibility becomes a particle and we become limited by our own beliefs.

Our true nature is so much more than our DNA could ever determine. Yet if we believe that we are merely a body governed by genes that run themselves, we will remain in conflict, expending our energy trying to protect ourselves from an ever-threatening environment, and the reality that we will manifest is one of ongoing conflict between wellness and dis-ease.

When the Tao is lost, there is virtue.
When virtue is lost, there is morality
When morality is lost, there is ritual.
Ritual is the husk of true faith,
The beginning of chaos.
Therefore the Master concerns herself
With the depths and not the surface,
With the fruit and not the flower.
She has no will of her own.
She dwells in reality
And lets all illusions go.

—*Tao te Ching, Chapter 38*

Illness is a process that begins much deeper than its surface expression and long before any of its symptoms become manifest. Rarely is the disease the problem, but the underlying misunderstandings it represents. If we see the manifestation itself as the problem, we usually waste our efforts attempting to alleviate something that isn't yet ready to resolve. We may lose not only our confidence in the ability to heal, but also our most powerful role in the healing process.

The radical grace that cures isn't available when we contract in fear because our methods are ineffective. Alternatively, instead of focusing on symptom resolution, we may view the illness as an invitation to begin an inner participatory quest of healing. Looking back we can inquire as to what types of signposts were offered along the way. Perhaps we became overcommitted to a particular task, leading to exhaustion, lack of appreciation of life, and poor eating habits, all of which can lead to the system breaking down. This is not a time to medicate but to take stock of physical and emotional needs. Treat the illness as a compassionate teacher. Vow to pay attention to its lessons, and change will be certain.

Real healing happens when we come back into alignment with the true nature of our Spirit. The most profound healing journeys often require some real soul searching, and a willingness to relinquish all that is not in accordance with the highest good. Yet it seems some are not yet ready for good health. Hippocrates said:

> If someone wishes for good health, one must ask oneself
> if he is ready to do away with the reasons for his illness.
> Only then is it possible to help him.

The Greek Father of medicine also coined the Latin phrase *primum non nocere*, the oath taken by doctors where they promise first and foremost to abstain from harming their patients. Yet we all know of someone, probably many people, who have been damaged by the pharmaceuticals they were prescribed. It isn't at all unusual for an individual to be on 10–15 different drugs to "treat" supposed abnormalities in their laboratory findings, and end up sicker and with more side effects than they had before going on them.

A great example of this is Stephanie, an extremely gifted and sensitive young woman who suffered a skiing accident in her twenties and broke her leg. Thankfully, her bones healed, but she remained in pain months after the accident, for which she was prescribed various pain relievers. As she became increasingly immobile and unable to work, she was eventually put on three different antidepressants, one on top of the other. While she used to be very active and health conscious, ten years later she was 80 pounds heavier and was on 12 additional medicines to help her sleep and treat anxiety, acid reflux, irritable bowel syndrome, fibromyalgia, diabetes, and a heart condition. She had a list of diagnoses that justified each medication she had been prescribed. While her leg wasn't particularly bothersome anymore, her whole body was in constant pain and she could barely get out of bed. She had consulted many specialists, but no one offered her anything but more medication; nor did any one physician look at the interactions and side effects of the drugs she was on. When we first met, she was puffy, sweating, and her lips and tongue were purple, as her liver was overwhelmed. Every single symptom she was experiencing was either directly caused by the medications she was taking or on their interactions. With the help of acupuncture, she was able to get off of all medications, drop the diagnostic disease labels, and resume an active and healthy life. But it wasn't easy, for there were many unacknowledged side benefits she received from her ailments. Over the years, she had developed a victim mentality, and had got stuck viewing herself as an invalid. She was receiving disability benefits, and had a loving, caretaking, albeit enabling husband who waited on her night and day. In order to heal, she had to recognize her reluctance to give all of that up.

Stephanie was a victim of a sick system that has lost its way. This is not to blame the medical system, for all societal constructs are manifestations of the mindset that created them. The brilliance of modern medicine and the compassionate gifts of its healing professions have become contaminated by the reliance on pharmaceutical management for most states of imbalance that could easily be resolved naturally, if one is ready to do away with the reasons for their illness. And the medical system serves and benefits from our reluctance to change. There is very little health or care in what has ironically become known as our "health care" system. Quite contrarily, the modern commercial medical industry is rewarded handsomely when we are sick, and thus has no real incentive to make us well. After all, who will purchase its medicines if we care for our own health and cure what ails us?

Every one of us is the product of a long line of ancestors who once knew how to allow healing to happen. How do we know this? Because we are here. Our great, great, great grandparents took the remedies nature provided and survived to produce offspring. It's in our cells. But somehow over the intervening centuries, these remedies, along with our innate wisdom, became downplayed or hidden out of sight. We forgot that if the right environment was produced, we would heal on our own. Private industries fabricated unnatural versions of nature's cures and convinced us we needed them, and they would be so good to sell them back to us.

So what might have led up to the madness of our present medical predicament? When did we cease honoring natural remedies that our bodies recognize, and turn our health over to an industry based on profit? Part of the answer lies in the early 1900s, when natural and herbal medicines were commonplace, and the progressive era of business expansion was just beginning to emerge with all its far-reaching consequences. While oil tycoon John D. Rockefeller (*How Rockefeller created the business of Western medicine*, 2019; *How John D. Rockefeller influenced modern medicine*, n.d.) was busily making billions of dollars extracting petrochemicals from the earth, the wealthiest American of all time recognized and turned his attention toward another tremendous profit motive which he then doggedly pursued. While full recognition of the toxic effects of petrochemicals hadn't yet surfaced, Rockefeller envisioned products derived from petrochemicals that could both capitalize on and revolutionize medicine, if only he could remove the public's reliance on archaic practices like healthy eating, herbs, bodywork, and bloodletting. He bought a German pharmaceutical company to get his foot in the medical door and, by ruthlessly funding his agenda, flung it wide open. In 1910, the Rockefeller Foundation hired Abraham Flexner, not a doctor but an educator with a bachelor of arts degree, on an investigative quest to redefine medicine. Flexner's report referred to antiquated practices like diet, nutrition, and naturopathy as quackery, and media campaigns were launched to discredit these unscientific and dangerous methods. Herbs were seen as especially troublesome, and were simply discounted as folklore and placebo. Meanwhile, they siphoned enormous amounts of money into large

universities. The Flexner report became a flimsy justification to change medical laws while Rockefeller used his money and reputation to persuade his
friends and contacts in Congress to push his agenda through.

Meanwhile, Rockefeller offered large grants to medical universities
with the agreement that they would be obligated to exclusively teach
allopathic medicine. Through Rockefeller Foundation funds, the entire
curriculum of medical education was restructured, dictating what and how
doctors were to be taught, removing all references to natural remedies and
replacing them with pharmaceutical intervention. The American Medical Association was endowed with unquestioned authority and became
the sole governing body required for allopathic licensure. Congress then
implemented this standard, which remains virtually unchallenged to this
day. Like carcinogenic petrochemicals, what began as a profit motive spread
like a cancer, and three years later, Rockefeller funded what would become
the American Cancer Society, which made it illegal to employ any natural
healing modalities in the treatment of cancer so all would have to rely
on surgery, chemotherapy, and radiation. The next year, the malignancy
attempted to spread to China, and in 1914 the Rockefeller Foundation
funded the China Medical Board to modernize the practice of medicine
in China, which fortunately mostly failed. But the effects of Rockefeller's
rampage remain alive and profitable today. Petrochemicals are utilized to
manufacture a plethora of safety devices and medical equipment such as
intravenous lines, syringes, heart valves, rubber gloves, hand sanitizers,
masks, and safety wrapping. Petrochemical-derived ointments, lubricants,
creams, gels, and suppositories have become a base for delivery of topical
drugs. Cough syrups, antibiotics, aspirin, and chemotherapeutic drugs are
synthesized from petrochemicals; in fact, most pharmaceuticals are made
using petrochemical polymers or are purified with petrochemical resins.
The pharmacopoeia the modern Western world wholeheartedly accepts is
riddled with toxins that we swallow unquestioningly because our highly
educated doctors prescribe them.

According to the Centers for Disease Control and Prevention (CDC),
today over 75 percent of hospital and clinic visits involve pharmaceutical
prescriptions. While it is not legal or ethical for doctors to write prescriptions for non-patients, over 85 percent of medical residents reported writing

prescriptions for relatives and friends. A typical medical doctor sees 25 patients per day, and writes 1.4 prescriptions per patient, which averages 35 scripts per day. If they work 300 days per year, that's 10,500 prescriptions annually per doctor. A common marketing strategy used by the pharmaceutical industry is to provide personal financial payments in cash and gifts to physicians. While it isn't legal, over two billion dollars per year is still paid to doctors by the pharmaceutical industry to increase prescription writing. Pharmaceutical reps provide free drug samples, while gifting fancy meals, trips, and other incentives to physicians who prescribe their drugs.

We may have overcome our disdain for cure-all snake oil remedies, but the pendulum has swung way too far the other way, where a century later there is a particular synthesized pharmaceutical to prescribe for nearly every recognized disease or laboratory abnormality. This has given rise to our present glorification of evidence-based medicine, built on the foundation of scientific materialism, which has been corrupted to the point that it has lost its validity. Now Big Pharma funds the blind research the entire system relies on for its truth, based on financial gain, not patient outcomes, and we simply cannot afford to believe their claims anymore. In 2022, there were almost 73,000 International Classification of Diseases (ICD) codes, and over 20,000 prescription drugs, with an average of more than 50 new prescription drugs approved for marketing by the Food and Drug Administration (FDA) each year.

This is no longer a system whose primary motive is health or wellness—it is industrial profits. It isn't that Western medicine is bad—far from it. But the institution has lost its way. Brilliant and well-trained doctors have hefty debts but are becoming so burned out they're leaving the field in droves. Insurance companies, FDA policies, and bureaucratic rules run pharmaceutical medicine far more than doctors do. Government, politics, economics, and medicine have all become intertwined in a sticky web that we agree doesn't work, but that nobody knows how to remedy. Instead of tearing the system down, let's begin at the bottom, where all true healing happens, and reach those who are ailing.

Just imagine what would happen if practicing physicians, the ones who have come into contact directly with suffering humanity, had some acquaintance with Eastern systems of healing. The Spirit of the East surges through every pore as a balm for all afflictions.

—Carl Jung

We all know and esteem the rich tradition from which East Asian medicine hails. While we must continue to respect the wisdom inherent in this system, we mustn't get our boots stuck in the past of our own tradition, either. Chapter 39 of the *Nei Jing Su Wen* states that *those who are good at speaking of antiquity must have made the junction with the present.* We live in a very different world today than our forebears and can embrace the tremendous advances modern biomedicine has offered. So in honoring tradition while making junction with the present, we can ask ourselves, what truths continue to recur? What do the wise healers of all time continue to rediscover? One of these perennial truths is that real cures come from within. Not within a pill or an herb, but within the infinite capacity of the human Heart to heal what ails us.

It is well understood in Chinese medicine that the Blood follows the Qi and the Qi follows the Mind. The Blood level could be viewed as the substance that Western medicine can scientifically examine, identify, and attempt to treat. Yet physical manifestations are most often effects, not causes. Thus, most pharmaceuticals address symptomatic effects, while the energetic causes remain hidden, at least until they show up with another manifestation later. It is not unusual, and often even expected, that prescriptions pile up later in life, as if chronic disease states are inevitable. It is simply not so. It is a result of a skewed perception from a worn-out paradigm that still chooses to believe that doctors are in charge of our health, laboratory analysis reveals where our sickness lies, and pharmaceuticals fix it. Even medications that are designed to address mental and emotional states are treating the branch rather than the root. While psychiatric conditions address "chemical imbalances," neurochemicals are produced by the state of the Heart-Mind, and the gut and its neurotransmitters are its reflections. The brain, which belongs to the Kidneys, projects the world through the Heart-Mind, which belongs to the Spirit. Therefore, all causes ultimately reside in the Heart. And so do their remedies. True healing is radical and necessarily involves a shift in consciousness.

Big Shen, the spirit of universal intelligence, is unitive; residing at all times as an indivisible whole that requires no healing. Yet as Big Shen localizes in an individual Heart-Mind, it generally perceives itself as a small separate body, and projects an experience of a large universe outside itself that could threaten it. This vibratory distortion creates anxiety in the Heart and tension in the body, resulting in a whole host of disease states.

The lowest energetic state of medicine treats diseases which have already manifested. Its whole premise is that one is already sick. It is based on fear of getting sicker or of dying, and being on the lookout for markers of disease, which are then labeled, solidified, and treated with particular synthesized pharmaceuticals that neither nature nor physiology recognizes, and therefore they are unable to restore harmony. Generally, patients are not asked to look within, evaluate their lifestyles, and make adjustments within their environments where they have a tremendous amount of control. This, the common prevailing medical paradigm, views human bodies as machines that are constantly moving toward entropy, disarray, or breakdown, unless they are intervened on, usually by whichever pharmaceutical is considered most appropriate.

The *Nei Jing* purports that low-level physicians find themselves salvaging what has already manifested in physical form, and treating what is already ruined. There is no need to change anything, just take this drug. And medical consumers dutifully go to their doctors because they believe that if they don't, they might just develop an illness which could kill them. This fear of becoming ill is an extremely stressful condition, which causes or exacerbates almost every disease state. And the fear-based cycle continues, as it generates money for the pharmaceutical industry that runs our medical system, followed by the insurance companies that cover their medicines, and finally the physicians who prescribe them.

The middle state of medicine is based on disease prevention. Eating natural, organic, whole foods, exercising, avoiding sugar, alcohol, and processed foods, and including sometimes quite expensive nutritional supplements to supposedly supercharge our cells is better for the gut, the blood, and organs, and will obviously improve some aspects of our physical functioning. While undeniably preferable to pharmaceutical management, this approach is still based on avoidance of physical disease and therefore fear, a relatively low energetic state which constricts the Pericardium. Based less on entropy than the lowest state, at best it maintains the status quo.

The highest state of medicine begins with the recognition that we are spiritual beings at one with the universe, and our physical, mental, and emotional states constitute the righteous Qi that determines the optimum functioning of the physical body. In this model, the Qi flows upward, redeeming Shen from Jing. The *Nei Jing* again asserts that superior physicians make it their prerogative to address imbalances before they have manifested structurally, preventing them from being in the position of having to treat disorders that have already progressed to the realm of the physical. At this state, we learn not just to prevent disease through what we consume and how we move our bodies, but to elevate our Heart-Mind to live in a state of unconditional joy and gratitude where we love our lives too much to allow sickness to enter. This, the highest energetic state that Eastern philosophic disciplines encourage us to attain, is predicated on a desire to know and live from our true nature, rather than following the lesser directive to escape from pain and move toward pleasure; running counter to our present conventional paradigm that attempts to alleviate discomfort at all cost. We were meant to evolve and overcome entropic tendencies in order to become better versions of ourselves.

We, especially in the Asian medical tradition, must cease glorifying conventional Western medical practices. Each system has its own respective strength. One is to treat the physical manifestations of disease; one is to transform energy. The founder of the School of Converging Chinese and Western Medicine, Tang Zhonghai, highlighted the distinguishing characteristics of the two traditions in his *Essential Meanings of the Medical Canons* with his famous dictum that Western medicine is good at visible configuration, while Chinese medicine is good at Qi transformation. And practitioners can only transform their patients' Qi to the extent that they have done their own inner integrative work to perceive from a state of oneness. While the Heart is the ultimate healer, compassion alone is insufficient to move the patient's spirits. The love must be infused with wisdom, strength, and trust, fruits of cultivation that have the power to overcome the negative forces of even the most doubtful minds.

As we go through different systems for which medications are prescribed, understand that we will be viewing from a medical paradigm which the *Nei*

Jing considers inferior. But we must start somewhere, and my hope is that we can relate to the visible configurations of pharmacological intervention through the patterns of Chinese medicine with a goal toward transforming Qi rather than merely maintaining homeostasis to help our patients arrive at higher states of integration.

We have very different health and disease landscapes today from when the *Nei Jing* was written. Our modern treatment methods have resulted in fewer deficiency diseases; however, we seem to have traded up for far more chronic excess disease states. While antimicrobials definitely helped alleviate many deaths due to bacterial infections, we are witnessing the emergence of ever more drug-resistant infectious disease agents. While at one end of the spectrum we are becoming more proficient at identifying and treating certain disease states, there seems to be a price to pay for thinking we can outsmart mother nature.

Thousands of years ago, the bark of the willow tree was found to relieve pain and lower body temperatures. From it was derived aspirin, one of the most commonly used drugs in the world. No longer the bark of the willow tree, but a synthetic derivative of its isolate, this chemical has also been found to lower platelets and inhibit prostaglandin synthesis. It wasn't until a chemist from Bayer was able to synthesize acetylsalicylic acid that it flooded the market, allowing the "acceptable" side effects of increased bleeding, stomach ulcers, potential damage to the liver and kidneys, and a rare type of brain swelling from mitochondrial damage. No Chinese herb would be allowed to stay on the market with such potential for harm.

Combined with the fact that pharmaceuticals are fabricated in laboratories, commercial prescription medications not only contain the active synthesized chemical, but they abound with toxic fillers, dyes, and expedients which can give rise to or exacerbate allergic reactions, sensitivities, intolerances, digestive disturbances, and even neurotoxic effects, whose iatrogenic origins remain mostly unrecognized and become reasons to prescribe yet other drugs to deal with their effects.

Elaine was an elegant woman in her eighties who dutifully followed her doctor's orders. She was taking eight prescription drugs for hypertension, Type II diabetes, mild depression, occasional heartburn, and various pain complaints. She also suffered from intractable diarrhea that caused her great embarrassment as she soiled herself almost daily. When she told her primary care physician what she was going through, he referred her to an allergist who diagnosed her with a wheat allergy. She removed all wheat from her diet, and the diarrhea lessened but did not abate. A year or two later she was diagnosed with a chocolate allergy, and although she lived for chocolate lava cake, mocha, and gluten-free chocolate croissants, she gave them all up. Doctor's orders. Once again, her symptoms temporarily improved. She tried not to complain about her dietary restrictions, but her greatest pleasures in life had been removed. Her daughter insisted her symptoms were most likely caused by one or more of the medications she was taking, and her doctor agreed to take her off Prilosec before she went on a cruise. Meanwhile, Elaine had decided to allow herself all the wheat and chocolate she wanted on this cruise. Much to her surprise, the diarrhea never returned. She didn't have a wheat or a chocolate allergy, but a sensitivity to Prilosec. It was the last place her doctor looked.

The *I Ching* tells us that life is nothing if not an ever-changing scenario where we are invited to find and live our highest truth according to the alternating patterns of nature. Yet we cherish what is known and predictable over the winds of change that urge us to expand and grow until we find our way home to ourselves. Drugs can help us through difficult times or keep us stuck in unconscious patterns without experiencing their consequences. If we take a drug for hypertension, for example, we will not have to lower our stress levels, change our diets, exercise, or learn to meditate. Antidepressants are often prescribed to cover up negative feelings about living in a rather insane world, a natural response to which would initially be to become depressed and anxious. Thus, we don't have to meet the discomfort, transform our Qi, and become more resilient in the face of whatever difficulty we encounter. Our motivation to remain comfortable can hinder our own growth. The effort to maintain status quo can cause unexamined psychological issues to become latent, manifesting later as physical disease processes.

The driving force behind most of our decisions is whether or not our actions will create relief from our discomfort or "Will this make me feel better?" Often people go to their doctors because in the face of whatever life challenges they are experiencing, they want to feel better. Attempts to make us feel better might provide relief, but can also create an ongoing cycle of feeding the need to feel better, and then better than that, all the time. Hence, feelings such as boredom or melancholy are taken to be wrong, and instead of learning to be present with whatever experiences life brings our way, we try to abate the discomfort with a drug, a drink, or some other distraction. This is the mindset that has to change, in all of us, in order to reduce reliance on pharmaceuticals.

We, in the healing profession, tend to operate from a perceptual field dominated by an ongoing process of diagnosing and treating. We look for what's wrong, and then try to remedy it. When patients come to us, they are generally feeling bad. They are often in fear, and pay us to find out what is wrong and fix it. While we may remedy their particular presenting ailment, we don't necessarily alleviate the underlying fear. In fact, we often feed the "feel better all the time" mindset instead of helping our patients increase the resilience of their righteous Qi so they may rise above whatever perceived evil Qi they are encountering. Sometimes our most well-intentioned means to fix what's broken is a form of violence. The *Tao te Ching* tells us that the world is sacred and can't be improved on, and that even well-intentioned violence always rebounds on oneself.

True curative medicine requires that we be rooted in spirit so we may move the patient's spirits in order to achieve an effect. No matter the acupoint, herbal formula, or other medical instrument, this will always be our goal. In fact, at this level, the tools we employ become less relevant. A simple touch or gesture can set the healing motion in place. As we venture through our study of pharmaceutical preparations, let's not lose sight of this fact. Healing does not require the use of drugs.

CHAPTER 2

Chinese Medicine Interfaces with Pharmacology

When the Tao is lost
There is medicine...

And between the two lies the great wisdom tradition of the Tao. Yet the way Asian medicine is taught today virtually drops practitioners into practice with very little experience and training, causing us to default to the mindset we grew up with. We memorize which points have what effects, and which herbs treat what diseases. Without appropriate supervisory guidance, some never graduate beyond this superficial approach. As such, many practitioners are not well versed in solid diagnostic skills, and treat diseases rather than the energetic patterns that cause them. As a profession, we are taught just enough biomedicine to understand basic allopathic approaches, but don't know how to incorporate them into Chinese medicine. We end up studying and practicing "adjacent medicine," where each remains within its own paradigm and where the two shall never meet.

We do not treat Western diseases with Asian medicine. It is my belief that we must translate Western disease states into Chinese medical patterns of imbalance, and do what we do best: treat the patient. In a recent doctoral class, a student asked me what the best herbal treatment for polycystic ovary syndrome (PCOS) was. It seems like a reasonably simple and innocuous question, and I could have answered that most classical PCOS presentations respond fairly well to modifications of Er Chen Tang. The question would have been answered in a minute, she would have felt as if she had the remedy in her tool box, and we could have moved on. But adjacent medicine doesn't work. True integrative medicine, on the other hand, does. We first had to lay the question aside and dig below the surface. I told her we don't treat PCOS. We treat individuals, and have to uncover the underlying pattern that caused the presentation which resulted in polycystic ovaries. Often, the sympathetic nervous system becomes dominant, and ovarian blood flow will be diminished. Sometimes Liver Qi stagnation predominates and there will be more adrenal involvement. In other cases, the Spleen Yang will be weak, predisposing to Dampness. Sometimes Phlegm covers underlying Blood Heat, both of which will have to be resolved. We have to understand what energetic patterns correspond with the pathophysiology before we can apply the tools of Asian medicine most effectively. The same student then asked why hypoglycemic drugs sometimes improve ovarian response. In order to answer this question, I had to explain the underlying patterns behind insulin resistance and glucose intolerance in the multi-endocrinopathy that impacts pancreatic, adrenal, and ovarian function. And then we had to take it one step further to understand the energetics of hypoglycemics. The real answer took about 60 times longer, but we had begun to approach true integrative medicine.

The focus of this work will therefore include strengthening your understanding of Chinese medical patterns and how they relate to the development of certain disease states rather than providing simple herbal or acupoint prescriptions for Western diseases. We will then apply the same approach to understanding the energetic effects of pharmaceuticals, without ever having to leave home base.

First, a little primer on the Western pharmaceutical approach, along with some correlations with Chinese medicine. The primary difference between medicines is basically that pharmaceuticals are synthetic, human-made imitations of isolated substances which have been found to induce or mute specific physiologic effects in the body to address symptoms caused by a recognizable disease process. Herbal medicines are found in nature, and are directed toward enhancing the body's underlying healing mechanisms.

Most disease states for which these substances are prescribed can fit into one of four basic categories:

- Infectious: viral, bacterial, fungal, parasitic
- Hereditary: genetics and hereditary disease states
- Physiologic: endocrine, neurologic, immunologic, or organ malfunction
- Deficiency: vitamin or mineral deficiencies

There are four basic categories of mechanisms in Western drug pharmacology:

1. The first involves stimulating or inhibiting production. Forteo is a parathyroid hormone drug, for example, which helps build new bone when bone loss is severe. Conversely, statins are prescribed to block the liver's production of cholesterol when laboratory values are seen to be pathologically elevated.
2. Reception involves how substances are received or absorbed in the body, either physiologically or pathologically. Many drugs inhibit how substances are received. The categories reveal their actions: calcium channel blockers, betablockers, angiotensin-converting-enzyme (ACE) inhibitors, gonadotropin-releasing hormone (GnRh) antagonists, dopamine antagonists.
3. Some drugs block reabsorption or impact elimination. Selective serotonin reuptake inhibitors (SSRIs) block reabsorption, increasing stimulation at synaptic connections. Cholestid binds bile acids in the intestines to increase their excretion.
4. Deficient substances are replaced: this includes vitamins and hormone replacement therapy, for example.

Research is scanty on how drugs and herbs interact, whether they are complementary or antagonistic. But we can make some correlations as we evaluate the pharmacodynamics and pharmacokinetics, which describe the absorption, metabolism, distribution, and elimination of drugs, as well as some interactions that might interfere with their intended mode of action.

- Absorption, which deals with how the body brings substances into the blood, is impacted by the route of administration. The solubility of the drug, the form of delivery (tablets, capsules, solution), the route of administration (oral, sublingual, topical, inhalation), and the rate of gastric emptying all impact absorption. Oral medications will be affected by our digestive capacity, and therefore rely on the strength of the Spleen and Stomach. If the Earth element is weak, the medicinal may need to be consumed more often to have the same effect. Some drugs are advised to be taken with food; some foods interfere with drug absorption, so must be taken on an empty stomach. With Chinese medicine, we take tonics with food, but in Western medicine, with the exception of vitamins, there are very few tonifying substances. Those that are taken on an empty stomach usually have some type of moving quality and go directly into the bloodstream without the interference of food. Certain medicines, like NSAIDs, antibiotics, narcotics, and cholesterol drugs, can cause stomach problems, however, and it might be suggested they be taken with food. The body is more acidic right after eating, and becomes more alkaline once the food is digested. Yang substances like amphetamines enhance gastric acid, so it is better to take them with food. Most absorption occurs in the small intestine, so herbs that increase peristaltic activity such as Da Huang or Huo Po will generally decrease absorption. Astringents like Wu Wei Zi and Shan Zhu Yu slow down intestinal motility and can therefore enhance absorption. Like milk slows down the absorption of drugs, sticky herbs like Da Zao and Sheng Di are like time-release medicines, and can also slow down absorption.

• Metabolism, according to Chinese medicine, is largely determined by the strength of the Spleen and Stomach. If the Spleen and Stomach are weak, the drug may need to be consumed more often to have the same effect. Western medicine views metabolic function as an activity of the liver, which determines the duration of efficacy of the drug. If liver metabolism is high, the dosage needs to be increased to maintain the same effectiveness. According to Chinese medicine, if the Liver is constrained and invades the Spleen and Stomach, vomiting or diarrhea may result, decreasing the efficacy of the drugs. Anticonvulsants like

Tegretol or Dilantin, intended to rid Internal Wind, speed up Liver metabolism. Alcohol slows it down. Drugs used to numb pain have a Dampening effect on the Liver, eventually making it more sluggish, but the Liver's initial reaction to the Dampness is to speed up, rebel, and metabolize quickly. If the Liver metabolism is slowed down, say because of alcohol use, the drug will stay in the system longer. Those with patterns of Damp Heat in the Liver may need to use lesser amounts of medicinals. Antibiotics and antifungals also reduce Liver metabolism. Minerals like Long Gu and Mu Li and antacids like Rolaids, Maalox, Tagamet, and Pepcid increase pH and thereby slow down metabolism. Gan Cao, on the other hand, increases Liver metabolism, so can move drugs out of the system faster, decreasing their efficacy and requiring higher dosages.

- Distribution describes how drugs are carried in the blood to different parts of the body. Some drugs bind to specific plasma proteins that render them inactive until they are released from the protein. These drugs are initially distributed to highly vascular organs like the brain, liver, and kidney; thereafter they are distributed to muscle, skin, and fat tissue. Anything that alters the separation from plasma proteins, like the majority of anti-seizure drugs, can affect drug distribution.

- Elimination of drugs from the system includes detoxification and excretion. Wood, Water, and Metal are the required elements that detoxify the body from pharmaceutical effects. The liver houses sophisticated enzymatic mechanisms to break down toxic chemicals that accumulate in fatty tissue. In phase one, toxic chemicals are converted into less harmful chemicals that are then conjugated in phase two to become water soluble substances that the kidneys can excrete through the urine. Metal then provides the route for release to the exterior via the breath, the skin, and the large intestine. Many drug-induced diseases are caused by the body's inability to fully break down or excrete the metabolites due to weak Zang Fu organs. This is especially true if one is on multiple pharmaceuticals. We also have to make sure that the medicinal has the appropriate exit route, whether it be through sweat, urine, or feces. Cold, Dampening drugs like analgesics can hamper elimination, which can then lead to autointoxication. Those who are deficient in Kidney Yang will have difficulty processing certain drugs, which can then cause Fire toxicity, which often manifests with a thick damp coating on the back of the tongue. They should take smaller dosages of herbs or drugs. Sprouts, watercress, celery juice, and daikon radish can assist with elimination. As we tonify the Kidneys and Liver and their function improves, so will elimination, as long as the bowels are functioning and urination is unobstructed.

Encapsulating portions of each of the above functions, from absorption to elimination, is the all-important role of the Small Intestine. The Minister takes its orders from the Emperor, whose job is to maintain the home of the Spirit, allowing in that which is pure and sending on that which is impure for this particular body-mind. This separation process is not just mindless sorting into a good pile and a bad pile, but represents the complex means by which the Heart's deep wisdom penetrates to allow certain substances to enter the Blood. The Small Intestine *receives* orders from the Heart, and then acts on them. While this is partially based on what enters the Stomach, the Small Intestine's selective permeability is meant to allow in that which resonates with the Heart. Anything that attempts to override this function, forcing artificial chemicals into the system which the body doesn't recognize as natural, can distort the impulses of the Heart and the gut-brain axis. This all important aspect of receptivity governs all bodily processes down to basic cellular function. For every physiologic action, there is a Yin (receptive) and Yang (active) component. First, the cellular receptors must be clean, open, and receptive to the incoming messages. Only then can the vital Yang movement be initiated. Sometimes our receptors are clouded because the Heart-Mind is deadened to its mandate from Heaven. The cells then cease to receive the messages, and have nothing to respond to. Agents should not be employed to force the movement until the portals are cleansed and the Empress is back on the throne, initiating orders that will keep the kingdom in harmony. Often when the portals are open, however, no medicines will be required.

Some drugs, toxins, and hormonal disrupters act by blocking or changing the configuration of the cellular receptor so the cell's natural function is subverted.

Depending on the molecule, this action could have a Dampening or Stagnating effect, which could manifest as a deficiency of whatever action (Yin or Yang) the physiologic process was meant to perform.

Those who are experienced in the true spirit of Asian medicine usually view the world through a different lens than their Western counterparts. We are somewhat bewildered that in order for medicine to be taken as "real," it must eliminate the placebo effect, or how our Heart responds to life. We acknowledge as fact that the care of the Spirit comes first; the Heart-Mind setting the tone for the Qi to follow, and then the Blood acts in accordance. It just doesn't make sense to put the Blood, or physicality, first, to which the Qi and Xin must adjust. Attempts to alter the body without including the Mind are doomed to fail. The Tao tells us if we go against the way of nature, the more tangled our delusional reality becomes and there will be consequences to pay.

We are referring to two different philosophical modes of thought, yet some basic comparisons can be made between basic East Asian medical definitions and their Western medicine counterparts, which we will use to evaluate the effects of pharmaceuticals. While our approach will vary for each category we cover, our goal will be to evaluate the medicinal in terms of organ system, Shen, Qi, Blood, Yin, Yang, Jin/Ye, the three levels of Qi, and/or the three treasures.

Vital substances and their correlations

Jing: Our essence, the very basis out of which we are made. Jing provides our genetic starting point: who we are before we think about who we are. Supplying the very foundation of who we are prior to conditioning, Jing gives rise to how we grow and develop through pre- and postnatal epigenetic influences. Jing governs reproductive and developmental potential as it expresses itself throughout the aging process. It includes the bone marrow's contribution to blood production.

Yin: Refers to dynamics which are interior, receptive, inferior, cool, and slow.

Yang: In contrast to Yin, refers to dynamics which are more exterior, active, superior, warm, and rapid.

Jin/Ye: Production and metabolism of body fluids (saliva, cerebrospinal fluid, tears, synovial fluid) and exocrine and endocrine function.

Blood: Derives from bone marrow and includes our nutritional status and oxygenation capacity. Blood carries the Shen, which includes our inner psychology and how we emotionally respond to ourselves, others, and the world.

Qi: Includes functions like adenosine triphosphate (ATP), ion transfer, neurological function, storage of cellular energy, muscular firing, and movement. Qi enters, exits, moves inward or outward, and ascends and descends.

Yuan Qi: Describes the level of our constitution, associated with the Kidneys, Bladder, and San Jiao. It is intimately associated with our genetics. Yuan Qi is our original Qi, similar to Jing, the precursor to metabolic function. For example, cholesterol production would be at the Yuan Qi level, while the active hormones estrogen and testosterone would be at the Ying Qi or Blood level. The steps of conversion from cholesterol to the hormones that act at the Blood level describe an important function of how Yuan Qi is transformed into Ying Qi. The underlying directives of Yuan Qi belong to the collective and thus will sacrifice the individual for continuation of the many.

Ying Qi: Provides the nutritional component of metabolic function, including the personal reflections of our inner substance and thought-based reality—how we digest the world. This includes Little Shen, carried in the Blood, that makes up our emotionality, and is associated with Stomach, Spleen, Heart, and Pericardium.

Wei Qi: Describes our defensive Qi, the protective functioning of our immune system. This energy tends to go outward toward the body surfaces, and also lines the gastrointestinal (GI) system. Wei Qi flows outside the blood vessels. It is associated with our defensive posturing in regard to our connections with the world and others and is especially linked with the Lung and Liver.

Shen: Include our very life force, vitality, psychology, consciousness, neurology, humanity's awareness of universal consciousness (Big Shen, accessed through the head), and our individual interpretation of the unitive source (Little Shen, located in the Heart).

Heaven: Symbolizes the highest cosmic principle, the unseen source, the origin of universal intelligence, represented by the invisible power of the vast sky, which is responsible for the myriad environmental and weather conditions, and the laws that govern the changing seasons of nature. Heaven is indistinct, but allows everything else to exist. We could say that Heaven even gives rise to the "God particle," the Higgs boson, responsible for granting mass to all other particles. The character for Heaven 天, Tian, shows a person with an added horizontal line on top, like a canopy that depicts our ability to connect with the realm of cosmic consciousness. The center of the brain, where the crown at Du 20 vertically meets Yintang horizontally behind the center of the eyebrows, is also where our brain's command post is, and where we are able to receive more subtle frequencies than those provided by the senses alone.

Response to pathogenic factors

Wind: Because Wind is changeable, it manifests as instability of physical metabolism, temperature dysregulation, transient symptoms, and tremors.

Cold: Results in decreased metabolism, hypothermia, and condensation of metabolic processes. This slow movement hinders Qi flow and can stagnate any humor, potentially leading to stagnation and stasis.

Heat: Produces enhanced movement and frenetic activity resulting in increased metabolism, fever, sweating, inflammation and rashes, rampaging cells growing out of control (cancer), agitation, and irritation.

Summer Heat: Often a combination of external pathogenic factors that tend to arise in hotter environments, overactive metabolic pathways, and dehydration in acute situations.

Dryness: Dehydration and other conditions which dry out the mucosal linings of the eyes, nose, mouth, the lower orifices, and the skin.

Dampness: Refers to a collection of fluid due to failures of fluid physiology. Dampness can result in edema or pooling; it gives rise to swelling, distension, and a sensation of heaviness. Dampness may result in electrolyte disturbances and endocrine congestion. Organisms like yeast and fungi tend to proliferate in Damp environments. Dampness often progresses to Phlegm if not resolved.

Phlegm: The accumulation of fluid that congeals in the mucous membranes, orifices, or cellular fluid. Phlegm may be visible or invisible, and its effects may be witnessed where consciousness is obstructed. Phlegm greatly hinders Qi movement and can give rise to tumorous congelations and angiogenesis.

Stasis: Refers to the tendency for Blood to clot or eventually congeal. This can be due to excess conditions that become chronic, or Blood deficiency where there isn't enough Blood to fill up the vessels and flow throughout the body, so it becomes like silt in a dry river bed.

Stagnation: Refers to a state where movement or metabolic functions have slowed down due to a certain internal pressurization. This can result in Heat, Cold, or Stasis. Pressurized or stagnant environments tend to produce Heat, which rises, exacerbating symptoms in the upper part of the body.

Latency: When the body-mind doesn't have the resources to metabolize a substance or process certain life experiences, it can be taken into storage, utilizing our available resources (Jing, Qi, Blood, or body fluids) to hold the substance at bay until we have the reserves available to metabolize it. If we don't develop the healthy reserves and state of mind to process the latent pathogen, it will often leak into circulation, producing bewildering symptoms of autointoxication and autoimmune conditions.

Responses to pharmaceuticals

Just like herbal medicines, pharmaceutical medicines impact the flow of Qi and Blood, although synthetic pharmaceuticals usually aim to override physiologic functions and rarely have fortifying effects. Caffeine may perk us up, but it doesn't tonify the Qi; it borrows Kidney Qi to stimulate the brain. We will rarely refer to their flavor, although some are distinctively sour, bitter, or salty. Since they are synthesized in a laboratory, most end up with a concentration that is difficult to quantify in terms the taste buds can distinguish.

Intended effects of the drugs initially depend on the state of the Stomach, Spleen, and Small Intestine's ability to digest, absorb, and utilize the medication. If these organs are deficient or obstructed, more medication is often prescribed to induce the desired effect; often resulting in iatrogenic diseases caused by the medication.

Some drugs induce Yang effects and raise the body temperature, produce sweating, or speed up metabolism; some induce Yin effects and cool down, blanket normal responses, or slow metabolism down. Some cause the Qi to ascend, descend, and move inward or outward. Some may obstruct the production of Jing or the flow of Blood.

We can also categorize the body's responses according to the three levels of Qi:

- Wei Qi responses include sweating, intestinal hyper-motility, allergic responses characterized by Heat, flushing, or swellings, and anaphylaxis. Like external weather impacts our state of mind, Wei Qi affects our moods.
- Ying Qi responses include Damp reactions like edema, those that impact the Blood level (red blood cells, white blood cells, and platelets), and systemic responses that impact the emotions or cause Shen disturbances.
- Yuan Qi responses impact the bones, the marrow, organs, and how we metabolize (Liver) and excrete (Kidney) the pharmaceutical agents. Yuan Qi belongs to the collective, and includes how our constitution is epigenetically programmed to produce our temperament.

Individual responses to medications

Paracelsus rightfully noted that *As a man imagines himself, so shall he be.* Place-bo-controlled studies, on which scientific method bases most of its research and conclusions, attempt to remove as much individual variability as possible. Lacking awareness of any mind-body connection, allopathic medicine blatantly and intentionally disregards the power of the Heart-Mind. Yet placebo, as we know, is capable of inducing profound therapeutic effects. The energy of hope lifts the Heart and heals. And the energy of despair constricts the Qi mechanism, rendering resolution more challenging. As my teacher Jeffrey Yuen has quoted of his grandfather, who took the onus off the diagnosis, *There are no incurable diseases; only incurable people.* The state of our mind matters. A lot.

When a medication is expected to provide relief, it tends to do just that. Patients who feel doomed to suffer generally do. Nevertheless, in spite of attempts to pigeon hole the general population, individual responses to pharmaceuticals vary greatly. Next to constitution and temperament that provide one's attitude toward healing, the most important consideration that determines how people will uniquely respond to a particular drug is what their underlying pattern of imbalance is—which is also likely to be responsible for the need for the prescription in the first place. For instance, those diagnosed with hypo*thyroid* will likely be prescribed one of the thyroid medications like Synthroid or Levoxyl, synthetic versions of thyroid hormone T4, thyroxine. Someone with a primary diagnosis of Spleen Qi deficiency will probably respond fairly well to the medication and perhaps their symptoms will be resolved. Someone else with Liver Qi stagnation may not fare as well, since the liver is responsible for converting T4, the inactive thyroid hormone, to its active form, T3. A person with Yin-deficient Heat may experience more side effects from thyroid hormone, which may exacerbate underlying Heat.

It is hoped that you will be able to utilize this material to see which individual patterns will respond better or worse to different pharmaceuticals, and will be able to improve overall physiologic function.

Basics of pharmaceutical analysis

This work is based primarily on a synthesis of my understanding of Western medicine and how to evaluate pharmaceutical and other substances into Chinese medical patterns. There are few written works on evaluating pharmaceuticals, although attempts to understand conventional medical approaches through an energetic lens have begun. Clare Stephenson (2017), in *The Acupuncturist's Guide to Conventional Medicine*, provides this simple and elegant six-step method for interpreting the energetic action of drugs in Appendix II in the back of the book:

1. How does the drug give relief of symptoms?
2. What is the Chinese medicine interpretation of the disease?
3. How does the drug alleviate disease in Chinese medicine terms?
4. What are the common side effects of this drug?
5. What is a simple Chinese medicine interpretation of the side effects?
6. Into what category of mode of action does the drug fit?

We can use these questions as a basis, and elaborate further until we understand how each drug or substance fits into a Chinese medical pattern diagnosis.

When we have answered these questions to our satisfaction, we should be able to define it by one of the diagnostic categories listed above. We may find it impacts the Yuan, Ying, or Wei Qi level. It may affect the distribution of body fluids. It may ascend or depress the Qi or invigorate Blood. It may inhibit or exacerbate Yin or Yang. When we have determined its energetic effects, we can enhance its action, utilize Chinese medicine as an alternative, or help alleviate some of its side effects.

As an exercise in practicing this process, we can utilize this method to evaluate vitamin A in terms of its Chinese medical energetics. While nature doesn't produce vitamin A in isolation, we can look at what we know of its effects:

- Vitamin A is a fat-soluble vitamin which is stored in and accumulates in the liver. It is found in fish oil, liver, egg yolks, and butter.

- It impacts vision, growth, cellular division, reproduction, and immunity, and maintains surface tissues and skin health.
- Being an antioxidant, it has a cooling effect.
- Deficiencies can give rise to skin diseases, risk of infections, and blindness.
- Overdose may result in joint and bone pain, visual disturbances, nausea, vomiting, skin sensitivity, hair loss, headache, raised intracranial pressure, and dry and itchy skin.

We can deduce, then, that vitamin A has a role in Kidney Jing (at the Yuan Qi level) becoming Liver Blood (at the Ying Qi level), as well as distribution to the Cou Li space (at the Wei Qi level). Conservative supplementation has more of a Blood tonifying effect, while at higher levels, it can become toxic and produce symptoms associated with Heat, rebellious (Liver) Qi, and the potential for Wind and Dryness. While dietary supplements may tonify as vitamin A does in low doses, rarely will pharmaceuticals result in tonifying actions.

The remaining chapters will utilize this same methodology, although I won't outline the steps with each pharmaceutical presented. As I'll be presenting only the most common drug classes in each category, if you wish to elaborate on any other specific pharmaceutical, you can use this process to evaluate other medicines or newer pharmaceuticals in the category. It is my hope that you, the reader, will take this work into the clinical field and really put it into practice.

CHAPTER 3

Microbiology and Antimicrobials

I am large, I contain multitudes.

—*Song of Myself*, 51

Walt Whitman, in *Song of Myself*, conveyed a spiritual truth so profound it can lead to our own awakening: we do indeed contain multitudes. While our Heart-Mind is capable of opening to vast celestial realms, our bodies are inhabited by trillions of viruses, bacteria, and fungi; in fact, these synergistic microbes outnumber our own cells ten to one. Viruses have altered our DNA and propelled our genetic evolution for millions of years. Fungi and yeast form an important role in harmonizing our gut microbiome. And bacteria, the foundation of our mitochondria, provide hundreds more protein encoding genes than do the human genome. They help us digest and absorb nutrients, they evolve our immune systems, and we literally could not survive without them. The myriad strains of pathogens that we house are as much "us" as the individual cells of our bodies are. Trying to kill one particular microorganism will disrupt the synergistic balance among the other microbes, and the complex physiology they help maintain.

Before antimicrobials arrived on the scene, infectious agents like viruses and bacteria ran their course, sometimes killing susceptible hosts. However, we hadn't yet become a germaphobic society, compulsively attempting to sanitize our bodies and sterilize our every environment. This cleanliness practice, once likened to godliness, not only weakens our immune systems, but encourages hardier germs. More robust cultures used to swim in ice cold water during the winter, get hot and sweaty during the summer, eat root vegetables without washing them first, sneeze and cough without barricading themselves, and share their eating utensils. In acclimating to the seasons and sharing their germs, their immune systems were able to combat most of the microbes they encountered.

Back to the *Song of Myself*, I will contradict myself in kind: we are not just what we think we are; yet how we experience life is based on what we think we are. If my identity and the orbit of my thought life is limited to my physicality, where I am threatened by organisms that are out to harm me, that will be my experience. If my sense of self is rooted in the macrocosm, I hold a much higher frequency and I am at peace. My true self cannot be harmed. Once again, the Heart rules.

The nature of Wei Qi

The nature of Wei Qi is that it allows the individual to interact with and become modified by environmental influences, meanwhile keeping the inner landscape safe and somewhat protected from what is outside. While Wei Qi provides a defensive function, it isn't meant only to separate us from but also connect us to our environment. We incorporate our environment into us as we harmoniously interact with the natural world in which we live.

Upright or Zheng Qi is a relative term which compares the strength of our own Qi to that of any potentially threatening pathogenic Qi. The *Nei Jing* tells us that *if righteous qi exists internally, evil cannot offend.* We can view this through the lens of the competitive survival of the fittest, where the only priority is "me vs. the other." This mindset reinforces the idea that the environment and its inhabitants are threatening, and our immune systems must respond and attack accordingly. Yet, the character for Righteous Qi, 正, shows Zheng as a process of correction where the Qi continues to be elevated to ever more righteous postures as we continue to evolve, through exposure, to become more just, integral, and upright. As this dynamic continues to be our primary focus, we are meant to become energetically higher than whatever external influences come our way as we remain safe. If we are following the true Way of our own evolutionary destiny, all exposures reveal that we are not limited isolated physical structures, but integral parts of a whole. This awareness raises our frequency along with the recognition that nothing can harm our true selves. No longer at war with a threatening world, we're inwardly tranquil, and relate to the whole world intimately as together we evolve into wider circles of acceptance and unity. We see ourselves more authentically as nature intended us to be, yet paradoxically less separate. Inner harmony and outer harmony become one. Yet if we are still conflicted internally, they can manifest in Wei Qi abnormalities. Conflicts surrounding our self-worth, which are carried in the Blood, can impact our sense of safety, protection, and defensiveness, in relationship to the world, and give rise to either heightened or diminished immune responses.

Wei Qi is an incredibly complex dynamic, whose production originates in Kidney Yang, the root of all warming functions of the body. This parallels the modern understanding that all immune cells are derived from common stem cells in the bone marrow. The Kidneys correspond to how we are rooted in and trust the essence of our very being. The San Jiao is also described as a source of both the defensive and constructive Qi. As San Jiao directs the distribution of Yuan Qi from the Gate of Life to the back Shu points, this evolutionary channel establishes our unique constitution.

When patients exhibit heightened sensitivity reactions, aggressive energy treatments can bring out any latent reactive Heat in the back Shu points and calm down immune hyperactivity. Wei Qi, being Yang, is said to circulate outside the vessels and body surfaces rather than within. But this doesn't relegate Wei Qi only to externally facing structures. The inner organelles of every cell are encased by membranous cell walls, which constitute their Wei Qi. These partitions function not only to separate, but also to allow routes of communication between cells as Qi enters and exits. Cellular function is primarily determined by the integrity and permeability of the cell wall, which can be stabilized with sweet and sour herbs. The Wei Qi of our skin and mucous membranes, epithelial tissue, and permeable intestinal walls determines how well they exchange and communicate. Their functioning is largely influenced by our deeply held beliefs, and how we view the world in relationship to ourselves. When we perceive the world as unsafe, it can weaken our Wei Qi. If we are at odds with the world, it can cause our epithelial tissue to become inflamed, in the form of Stomach Heat, evidenced by the appearance of a red tongue, lips, and gums, as well as the development of ulcers.

Wei Qi is derived from Ying Qi, pertaining to the Stomach and Spleen, and is distributed by the Lungs. Ying Qi, which is located within the vessels, must also be warm to prevent the Wei Qi, which occupies the exterior, from escaping. Wei Qi is described as warm, fierce, slippery, and rapid, and is concentrated in the external surfaces of the gut and orifices. This includes the glandular structures of the tonsils, adenoids, Peyer's Patches, and Appendix. Wei Qi initiates the gut's peristaltic movement (a Yang Ming function), fills the skin, fattens the interstices, and manages the opening and closing of pores and, to a certain extent, sphincters. The Lungs direct the Qi, descend Qi to the Kidneys, and diffuse Wei Qi to the surface. The strength of this function can be assessed through feeling the right Cun pulse. The Lung position should have superficial strength—as you raise your finger to the surface, the pulse should lift and spread, which measures the Lung's ability to disperse Wei Qi. The strength of the Lung Qi is also related to the vigor of the Spleen Qi and Kidney Qi; the communication between these three Zang organs should be checked on the right pulse. Jing tonics Lu Rong and He Shou Wu nourish the marrow to help tonify the Qi and Blood. Herbs that tonify the Kidneys can decrease immunoglobulin E (IgE) in atopic asthma, and regulate T cells.

The organs responsible for postnatal energy production—Kidney, Stomach/Spleen, and Lungs—are often deficient when Wei Qi is weak; these same organs deal with the accumulation of Dampness and Phlegm, which often manifest when Wei Qi is obstructed. Symptoms of deficient Wei Qi include fatigue, increased environmental sensitivity, decreased sweating, and hindered peristalsis.

The interstices circulate Wei Qi, which is associated with San Jiao's control of the waterways. This Cou Li space between the skin and muscles diffuses Wei Qi, which allows Jin fluid to be released in the form of sweat. The entering and exiting of Qi is governed by the pectoral Qi in the chest, Zong Qi. The circulation of Wei Qi begins at UB1 at the inner corner of the eye where it emerges at sunrise, allowing the Hun to extend outward so we can see what we project; it circulates through the Yang channels 25 times during the day, peaking around noon. At sunset, the Wei Qi enters the Kidneys and circulates 25 times through the Yin channels at night, where there is a grand meeting of the Yin, total emptiness, associated with the pure potential of San Jiao, represented by the hexagram of six Yin lines (☷), around midnight. As it says in the *Nei Jing*:

> Huang Di asks Qi Bo why the elderly don't sleep well. Qi Bo says: The strong have an exuberance of Qi and Blood, they have fatty flesh and muscles, their pathways of Qi are unimpeded, and their Ying and Wei are without irregularity. Thus they are energetic by day and sleep at night. As for the old, their Qi and Blood are diminished, their flesh and muscles are withered, their pathways of Qi are astringed, *the Qi of the five viscera are in conflict with one another*, Ying Qi is decrepit and scant, and the *Wei Qi harasses the interior*. Thus by day they are not energetic and by night they cannot sleep.

Once again, Huang Di and Qi Bo have beautifully described how unresolved internal conflict between Ying and Wei Qi, which tends to worsen with age, produces symptoms like insomnia, chronic inflammatory diseases, and autoimmune reactivity. This perfectly parallels the modern Western understanding that the immune system is weakened through age, fear, stress, dietary and environmental toxins, and isolation. A healthy immune system at any age is not only strong, but wise, able to discern what is friend and what is foe, leaving healthy cells and tissue alone. Treatments to strengthen Wei Qi may need to fortify the Qi of the Kidney, Spleen/Stomach, and/or Lungs, but may also need to calm down overactivity in the form of Heat, Stasis, Dampness, or Stagnation so it can circulate throughout the system smoothly. Here we are simultaneously strengthening the immune system while reducing any autoimmune overactivity. When we mindfully allow our systems to become challenged by external influences, our upright Qi becomes stronger. This not only pertains to meeting pathogenic factors, but meeting all of our life's unresolved conflicts to alleviate internal threats as well. Harmonized Wei Qi is in calm and alert recognition, silently inactivating potential harmful influences; it is strengthened through exposure, developing resilience to its ever-changing environment, overcoming internal sources of stress and not wasting its Qi fighting external or internal fights that can't be won. The Way is simple, although it isn't always easy or commonplace to practice such radical non-resistance.

The thymus gland's production of T lymphocytes is a great example of how our immune system evolves. The thymus gland is part of our adaptive immune system; it is located above the heart and pericardium, between the lungs, and protected by the sternum. When we are exposed to environmental factors, the thymus gland educates white blood cells by encoding our reaction into a T-cell that remembers how to respond to infected or cancerous cells. Very active early in life, the thymus gland produces T lymphocytes, cells that survey the rest of the system, distinguishing our own body cells from those that are seen as foreign or potentially dangerous. It protects self, ousts invaders, and remembers each encounter, always becoming more efficient if we heed its righteous movement. The thymus gland itself, by design, becomes less active as we age unless we are revitalizing it through Jing-cultivating longevity practices. As we mature, we become less reactive to insults, but the thymus gland also makes hormone-like substances essential for immunoregulation during aging. This represents how Zong Qi, the pectoral Qi associated with Metal and Fire at the interface between the neuroendocrine and immune systems, encodes the Heart so that Wei Qi gets smarter as we mature, rather than weaker or more defensive. Eastern traditions link this with the *higher heart*'s unconditional love of all things. When we have learned our inner lessons and resolved our inner conflicts, we can be freed of the ego, where our energy becomes directed toward spiritual growth and transformation. Tending to this powerful junction of Lung/Heart energies may represent our highest destiny—letting go beyond the small self that needs to be defended, into a unitive recognition of love where Big Shen resides. Our insides become less reactive to our outsides when, through our own conscious evolution, we see there is no real division. Thymic weakness can be associated with vulnerability of the Lungs and feelings of inadequacy. Remember that the Lungs are strengthened by letting go, not by holding on to defensive posturing. As we evolve, we gain in integrity and harmony as we expand to become the web of nature herself. As such, we experience ourselves as less and less separate, being made up of our environment more than distinctly cut off from it.

Qualities of pathologic Qi

Perverse Qi is not visible to the naked eye, but airborne factors are said to be carried through the Wind. The insubstantiality of unseen evils can include climatic factors like seasonal affective disorder. The low mood associated with it engenders a state of disdain, which in turn can generate immune reactions. Around 600 CE, Chao Yuanfang's *Origin of the Etiology of Disease*, a text of empowerment, taught us that all we ever need is contained within, if only we pay attention. Very little acupuncture or herbal medicine was prescribed, but instead focused on Tao Yin exercises, dietary recommendations, and the importance of tending to the messages received from nature. The 18th-scroll of the text provided a useful illustration of how to relate to parasitic microorganisms no matter the origin. It says that we're each born with 80,000 inadequacies and imbalances that dispirit or violate us. These "corpse worms" were seen as resident demons or deities (depending on how you relate to them) which remain dormant in the bowels until the correct environment awakens them. This doesn't mean we shouldn't awaken them; it is part of our destiny to meet environments that will transform us. There are nine types of worms, associated with nine fundamental lessons or heart pains, which are also called the Nine Palaces in Taoist alchemy, where these themes can be transcended. When these issues are unconscious and remain unresolved, they propel the motor that drives self-will. Our most compelling yet troubling life issues usually have to do with states of health, relationships, having enough/finances, prosperity/reputation, creativity/children, global/travel, professional knowledge, wisdom of knowing one's true self, and home/sense of completion.

These invisible organisms tend to thrive in sweet and fermented environments, and also represent the psychological themes that feed them—our three major sources of attachments and addictions:

- Those that pertain to the Lower Jiao have to do with physical lust, including desires for physical security and survival instincts.
- Those of the Middle Jiao play out our desires for comfort, satiation, and gluttony.
- Those of the Upper Jiao are our most glorified attachments—spiritual greed or ambitious pursuits where we desire to see ourselves as more elevated than our peers. These are actually highly prized in our society.

These pathogens aren't really evils, but may be seen as strict teachers. Yet they aren't innocuous; they may have the effect of gnawing away at and consuming our Essence until our curriculum is met and its lessons are learned. The microorganisms we can see are referred to as Chong; those we can't see Gu; those which produce bizarre behavioral changes Gui; and the malevolent ones that intend to cause harm are referred to as Mo. These don't imply that some are good and some are bad; they describe a spectrum of how the Shen recognize and respond to these visitors as a part of our curriculum. Very few of us are enlightened enough to welcome these pesky critters lurking in the depths as they come out of hiding to create symptoms that disturb our present state of equanimity. But like all symptoms, they can be read as signposts we are meant to decipher on our evolutionary journey and ultimately overcome. When we tune within and befriend them, recognize where we are out of alignment, and have the courage to change our internal landscape instead of medicating it, they settle down and leave on their own accord. If we only target the symptoms or attempt to kill the bugs, we haven't learned the lesson that will shift consciousness and its inner environment. They'll be back again, usually with a heightened learning experience next time.

These organisms help us grow, challenge us to evolve, and, yes, can sometimes overwhelm our systems and challenge our present state of health. Yet when our only focus is to annihilate them, we stay at the energetic level where they penetrated our defenses in the first place. There are two strains of thought regarding pathogenic factors: 1) kill the bad and return to "normal" or 2) raise our own Qi so that our own immune systems work it out within, followed by self-correction, and evolving so that our environment continues to become less threatening. You might be thinking, why not do both? Valid point, as long as a higher state of consciousness guides your actions. And that higher state of consciousness doesn't view anything as bad.

Remember that fear inhibits the immune system by contracting and descending energy downward, thus obstructing Wei Qi's distribution to the surface, as well as preventing our ability to strengthen our upright Qi and evolve. When we try to protect ourselves from pathogens (including those things within us that we perceive as evil), our resistance actually gives them power. Instead of resisting fear, we have to witness how it controls us; only then can we get beyond it. Perhaps you've had the experience of riding on an airplane surrounded by strangers. A neighboring passenger might be coughing and sneezing, and the "normal" response is to become defensive, covering your nose and mouth, especially if they haven't covered theirs. As soon as we fear we might get sick, we become stressed, our energy contracts, and immunity lowers. Then experience proves our suspicion and we become ill.

Instead, you might want to try an experiment and allow the germs to spread, as germs are meant to do. The real challenge is to observe what's going on inside, rather than outside. Wind calls forth change, and often external Wind meets internal resistance. If we contract in fear, we can't respond to the winds of life that lead us toward our destiny. Not only does fear weaken Kidney Qi, it contracts the Pericardium and inhibits the Heart's expansion. When noticing a tickle in your own nose or throat, don't tell yourself you are going to get sick, or tell yourself that you aren't going to get sick. Instead, focus on the fact that your own immune system is responding appropriately to the environmental changes life has brought your way. This calls forth more trust, which tonifies the Kidneys, and the righteous Qi to meet whatever external factor is present to guide you on your way. It's all consciousness. *If righteous qi exists internally, evil cannot offend.* This statement is either fact or theory; we either live it or we don't.

Infectious diseases

Pestilent Qi describes the behavior of an actual infectious agent of potential harm. While they are not visible to the eye and therefore fall into the category of Gu, when viewed microscopically, they become Chong, now visible. If they hide out and wreak havoc on the psycho-neuro-immunologic system, they may be referred to as Gui, and if they make the patient seem crazy or mentally disturbed, they have crossed into the threshold of evildoing, and are known as Mo. But remember, it is our conscious response to them that determines how they will move through our system.

External pathogenic factors (EPFs) can cause acute, chronic, and latent effects in the body. We define the nature of the pathogen by the energetic response it induces.

Pestilent factors enter the body and invoke exterior Wei Qi responses at the Tai Yang stage. The use of antimicrobial agents and medications to reduce their symptoms is thus classified as acting on the Tai Yang stage. Some of them, like antihistamines, are attempting to clear Heat, which suppresses Wei Qi's Yang reaction. This process may reduce Heat reactions, but also suppresses Tai Yang's ability to expel the pestilent factor, which can then become latent, only to emerge later. In fact, epidemiological studies of those who take antihistamines for long-term allergic reactions show a greater chance of developing immune compromised conditions and cancer.

Antimicrobial drugs to combat infectious diseases

As we discuss the drugs that kill the germs, notice that all of these "anti"-medicinals block the metabolic pathways of organisms in our body.

Viral pathogens require a host in which to replicate; they are generally short lived, most impact the upper respiratory tract, and resolve on their own. While viruses are usually considered Cold, which constricts and draws inward toward the solid Zang organs, they often manifest with Heat symptoms. We need this Yang response, contained in Tai Yang (UB/SI), to move this Cold to the exterior. This correlates to the first level of entrance according to the six divisions. Yet viruses can move deeper into the Constitutional level (DNA) via RNA replication. They can also turn off our internal security alarm systems and lie dormant in Cold environments, flaring up when aggravated. They can also show up as Damp febrile diseases with thick, sticky phlegm. Viruses have been and remain a fact of our evolutionary development. About 10 percent of our DNA is viral, which has mutated to become benign, friendly, and even beneficial—sometimes necessary for our very survival in changing times. We can't ever be free of viral pathogens; like many other pesky irritants we'd rather alleviate, it's often better to accept their presence and live with them harmoniously, where they can be incorporated into our systems to help us evolve, and/or become inactivated by our righteous Qi.

Over-the-counter cold medications

Most of the medications on the market only address the symptoms of viruses. They do not stop the progression of or hinder the virus at all, they merely mute our awareness of what's going on internally, which only Dampens our own Qi mechanism. I was recently at a neighbor's house whose TV was on during the evening news. The big headline of the day very dramatically and loudly pronounced that pharmacies were *running out of medication!* After an agonizing build-up, when the piece finally played, the announcer portrayed the serious and immediate threat of three deadly viruses running rampant and out of control—Covid-19, respiratory syncytial virus, and the flu—and that the public was in grave danger because the drug manufacturers weren't keeping up with the demand for medication. The camera panned along the cold and flu aisles at a local drug store whose shelves of over-the-counter decongestants, antihistamines, and cough suppressants were nearly empty. That's it. Hardly any Robitussin, Sudafed, or Benadryl left, or any of the myriad medications that combine them with pain relievers like NyQuil or Theraflu. I was initially eye-rollingly amused by the hype, and pictured the mass hysteria as everyone ran out to purchase any remaining cold medicine, just in case. Then I thought, how sad it is that this type of panic is taken as normal, and that our media-driven view of health is nothing but stress, the build-up of danger and fear, in this case of not being able to alleviate the symptoms of a cold. So let's bring a logical response into view and evaluate the symptoms of a typical Wind-Cold invasion so we can see how cold medicines impact its progression.

As respiratory viruses enter the nasal passages and begin to replicate, the immune system responds, in part, by sending immune mediators like neutrophils (Tai Yang) and eosinophils (Yang Ming) to defend the local site of entrance. This is how the Wei Qi diffuses Yang fluids to protect the exterior, as the Stomach ascends thin fluids to the upper orifices. First, B cells are activated from the bone marrow to make IgE antibodies that activate an emergent response, and these are then picked up by mast cells as they travel to the nasal mucosa and spew forth histamines. These hot little signaling molecules arouse us and send messages between cells. They increase blood flow and vascular permeability so white blood cells can reach the local area and go to work inactivating the invader at the tissue site. In response, the eyes may become inflamed and itchy, and as the nose becomes agitated, sneezing may ensue to assist in expelling the irritant. The mucosal tissues swell, decreasing the air passage through the nasal canal, potentially stagnating the Qi and causing pressure in the sinuses. Local inflammation can then trap the fluid as Dampness and Phlegm. Nasal discharge causes the nose to run, and excess mucus may drip down the back of the throat causing bronchial reactivity and the development of a cough. As Kidney Yang activates the Wei Qi, body temperature rises to shift the internal environment, and Heat helps expel the Cold invader.

These symptoms are, no doubt, annoying, but they are natural and necessary. Before medicines were developed to reduce the symptoms of a cold, we typically drank lots of water and juice, ate soups rich in bone marrow and vegetables, flushed our sinuses with salt water, used steam inhalation with essential oils, put warm compresses over our sinuses, and stayed in bed. We freed up the flow, rather than stagnating it. Some cultures took cold plunges in water to activate a Tai Yang response at the beginning of a cold. Our immune systems went to work, and we recovered. When we block the symptoms, we may be able to function pretty much as if we were not ill. But when we're sick, we're sick. We are meant to have fevers, runny noses, coughs, sore throats, vomiting, and diarrhea. Some studies have shown that our attempts to alleviate fever, congestion, cough, and runny nose actually prolong the duration of the illness. Some are Cold and Drying, others over-stimulate. What these all have in common is that they interfere with the body's natural Wei Qi responses.

Cough suppressants like dextromethorphan suppress the cough reflex in the brain in response to throat and bronchial irritation. Lung-astringent qualities can hinder the Lung's ability to diffuse and clear mucus. The down bearing action of the suppressants also act on several neuroreceptors in the brain implicated in depression, potentially causing dizziness, and drowsiness.

Expectorants like Guaifenesin help thin the mucous secretions that are difficult to expectorate, similar to phlegm-softening herbs. Side effects include constipation, headache, dizziness, and fatigue, and while they increase renal clearance of phosphate and uric acid, the eventual drying effect can also result in the formation of kidney stones. We can also use Xiao Xiong Tang to expel accumulated Phlegm in the chest.

Decongestants like pseudoephedrine or phenylephrine act by constricting the blood vessels in the nasal passages to provide relief from pain and pressure caused by the swelling nasal mucosa. But as the blood vessels narrow, fewer immune cells can arrive at the site of entrance, stagnating the Qi and Blood locally. Like Ma Huang, ephedra-based preparations are warm, pungent, and slightly bitter, but unlike Ma Huang, they don't induce sweating. These drugs have a stimulant effect, and the increase in Yang Qi can raise blood pressure and affect the heart rate, potentially causing anxiety and insomnia, much like rising Liver Yang can harass the Heart. The Yang action can also induce drying effects, which impacts fluid metabolism and reduces the Jin fluids required to flush the pathogen out.

Antihistamines block the body's production of histamine. There are two primary classes of histamine receptors: H1 receptors that drive vasodilation, bronchoconstriction, and nociception, which have more of an effect on the respiratory mucosa and skin; and H2 receptors that occupy the surface of gastric parietal cells, stimulating gastric acid secretion and motility.

Antihistamines
H1 antihistamines
There are two types of H1 antihistamines used for respiratory and dermatologic reactions:

- First-generation antihistamines (which cross the blood brain barrier and thus make the user drowsy), such as:
  - Diphenhydramine (Benadryl)
  - Doxylamine (Unisom)
  - Hydroxyzine (Atarax, Vistaril)
  - Tripelennamine (Pyribenzamine)
  - Carbinoxamine (Ryvent)
  - Bromazine (Ambrodil, Deserol)
  - Clemastine (Meclastin)
  - Pheniramine (Avil)
  - Chlorphenamine and dexchlorpheniramine (Chlor-Trimeton, Piriton, Polaramine)
  - Brompheniramine (Dimetapp)
  - Triprolidine (Flonase, Actidil, Myidil)
  - Dimetindene (Fenestil)
  - Chlorcyclizine (Diparalene, Mantadil, Pruresidine, Trihistan)
  - Cyproheptadine (Periactin).

- Second-generation antihistamines (which don't cross the blood brain barrier and cause less drowsiness), such as:
  - Bilastine (Blexten, Fortecal)
  - Cetirizine (Zyrtec)
  - Desloratadine (Aeries)
  - Ebastine (Evastin, Kestine, Ebastel, Aleva, Ebatrol)
  - Fexofenadine (Allegra), ketotifen (Zaditor)
  - Levocetirizine (Xyzal)
  - Loratadine (Claritin)
  - Mizolastine (Mizollen)
  - Quinenadine (Rupafin)
  - Terfenadine (Seldane).

While effective at reducing runny noses, sneezing, watery eyes, itching, and hives, these drugs can also dry out the precious Jin/Ye, leaving parched tissue in their wake. This can thicken mucus in the respiratory tract and make it more difficult to expectorate. In addition to drying fluids, which suppresses the necessary fluid discharge, they can also suppress the Wei Qi's Yang response. When we suppress the Wei Qi response instead of allowing it to move up to clear Wind in the eyes and nose, the suppressed Wei Qi can move inward and down to Yang Ming, where patients may experience symptoms of Heat, and Dry sensory orifices. They can also reduce the passage of urine, increasing the likelihood for urinary tract infections. These drugs are Cold and variably sedating, which is why they can produce drowsiness, brain fog, and confusion. Their Cold nature suppresses Wei Qi's Heat response, but also can dampen, causing the pathogen to linger. Long-term use of antihistamines can result in symptoms of Heat like constipation, which impacts the pure fluids and dries out the sensory orifices. We need to encourage generating fluids, with formulas like Ge Gen Tang, and herbs like Gui Zhi, which can assist the normal Wei Qi response.

Some antihistamines like diphenhydramine (Benadryl) also have anticholinergic properties that block the neurotransmitter acetylcholine, which is essential to learning, memory, attention, and alertness. This can manifest as loss of Shen Ming to the Sea of Marrow, and has accordingly been shown to increase the likelihood of developing Alzheimer's dementia.

While we are on the subject of antihistamines, we will take a little detour to the gut, which is chock full of Wei Qi. Physiologic Stomach Fire in the form of hydrochloric acid must be countered by sufficient Stomach Yin, represented by the adequacy of stomach mucosal lining. If this Yin/Yang pair is not harmonized, heartburn and gastro-esophageal reflux symptoms may result. Our approach can be to clear excess Fire with bitter cold herbs like Zhi Mu and Shi Gao, while nourishing fluids with herbs like Geng Mi, but we must take care to restore the physiologic Stomach Fire and bring stomach acid back up.

H2 antihistamines

H2 blockers like famotidine (Pepcid), cimetidine (Tagamet), nizatidine (Axid), and ranitidine (Zantac) are antihistamines that act on the gut to block release of physiologic Stomach Fire, required to digest Gu Qi. While excess Stomach acid can be associated with Yang Ming Heat, inhibiting hydrochloric acid production can temporarily reduce symptoms, but they are not curative and also interfere with the absorption of certain nutrients that require acidic environments. Long-term use can cause the Stomach Fire to be diverted to the Lung or Liver, and may manifest with Tai Yang or Shao Yang stage signs and symptoms.

Proton pump inhibitors

Proton pump inhibitors like omeprazole (Prilosec), esomeprazole (Nexium), lansoprazole (Prevacid), rabeprazole (Aciphex), pantoprazole (Protoniz), and dexlansoprazole (Dexilant) also block the production of stomach acid, which diminishes the Spleen's transportation and transformation functions. This creates an environment conducive to Damp accumulation, and can diminish absorption of essential nutrients like vitamin B12. Their use also can interfere with bile acid production, concentrating and congealing bile, and creating Cold in the Gallbladder. Long-term use can produce Phlegm obstruction, and can hinder the proper functioning of the stomach's parietal cells, sometimes even damaging them permanently. Bai Hu Tang can clear excess Stomach acid and generate fluids. Adding Ren Shen can help strengthen the Spleen, and Wen Dan Tang can address Gallbladder issues.

Antiviral drugs

- Abacavir, acyclovir, adefovir, amantadine, ampligen, amprenavir (Agenerase)
- Atazanavir (Efavirenz/Emtricitabine/Tenofovir)
- Baloxavir morboxil (Xofluza), bictegravir/emtricitabine/tenofovir alafenamide (Biktarvy), boceprevir, bulevirtide
- Combivir (Lamivudine/Zidovudine)
- Daclatasvir (Daklinza), darunavir, delavirdine, emtricitabine/tenofovir alafenamide (Descovy), didanosine, docosanol, dolutegravir, doravirine (Pifeltro)
- Edoxudine, efavirenz, elvitegravir, emtricitabine, enfuvirtide, ensitrelvir, entecavir, entravirine
- Famciclovir, fomivirsen, fosamprenavir, foscamet
- Ganciclovir (Cytovene)
- Ibacitabine, ibalizumab (Trogarzo), idoxuridine, imiquimod, inosine pranobex, indinavir
- Lamivudine, letermovir (Prevymis), lopinavir, loviride
- Maraviroc, methisazone, moroxydine
- Nelfinavir, nirmatrelvir/ritronavir (Paxlovid), nevirapine, nitazoxanide, nervier
- Oseltamivir (Tamiflu)
- Penciclovir, peramivir (Rapivab), pleconaril, podophyllotoxin
- Raltegravir, remdesivir, ribavirin, rilpivirine (Edurant), rimantadine, ritonavir
- Saquinavir, simeprevir (Olysio), sofosbuvir, stavdine
- Taribavirin (Viramidine), telaprevir, tebivudine (Tyzeka), tenofovir alafenamide, tenofovir disoproxil, tipranavir, trifluridine, trizivir, tromantadine, truvada, umifenovir
- Umifenovir (Arbidol)
- Valaciclovir (Valtrex), valganciclovir (Valcyte), vicriviroc, vidarabine
- Zalcitabine, zanamivir (Relenza), zidovudine

Antivirals subdue the spread of viruses rather than killing them. Different mechanisms include suppressing their ability to infect and multiply in our cells, or inhibiting molecular interactions required for their replication, thereby shortening the duration of the illness. Their greatest effect is produced when given right at the onset of the infection to reduce the severity of complications in susceptible individuals. While most antivirals target viral proteins, some target human proteins. As they disrupt our system, they can induce side effects like dry mouth, cough, diarrhea, fatigue, headache, insomnia, and joint and muscle pain. Those which have an effect on the epithelial cells of the kidney can cause renal failure. Their inhibitory effects on our own immune cells can lower immunity, especially for those who have been on them for prolonged periods of time.

We can make a sweeping generalization and say that repressing the ability to spread and reproduce is an energetically Cold effect. We also know that Cold tends to decrease metabolism and induce latency. And it follows that antivirals also tend to obstruct the free flow of Qi, cause counterflow Qi, and produce dryness. Our treatments, of course, will be to restore the free flow of Qi, tonify Qi, Yang, and Yin, stimulate thin fluids to the face (St 42), restore the descending of Qi, and astringe the intestines if appropriate (although we do not astringe the intestines if diarrhea is caused by a pathogen). Further, we will be identifying the nature of the Wind invasion and help release the exterior with formulas such as Yin Qiao San for Wind Heat or Ren Shen Bai Du San for Wind Cold so that the immune system can resolve the virus on its own. Acupuncture can stimulate a stronger Wei Qi response, reduce cough, and treat headaches and nasal congestion. Neurological symptoms arising from long-term post-viral complications are often treated by utilizing the Gallbladder, in part, to reach the brain and clear the orifices.

When Wind Cold is not resolved, it may give rise to Wind Heat or Wind Damp. The Yang Qi and Wei Qi are still trying to fight off the invader, which gives bacteria and fungi the opportunity to proliferate. Generally, when the immune system hasn't been able to clear the virus at Tai Yang, it may develop into a bacterial infection where Heat moves into Yang Ming, as Heat tends to go to the Fu organs. If the bacterial invasion is treated with antibiotics which give rise to Dampness, it increases the likelihood to develop a fungal terrain where yeast likes to proliferate. Dampness then tends to go to the various Fu, perhaps giving rise to Bi syndrome and autoimmune conditions like rheumatoid arthritis.

Vaccinations

Most vaccines work by injecting an inactive infectious agent directly into the bloodstream to stimulate an immune response without developing the disease. While there has been much controversy over recent vaccinations, Chinese medicine was the first to experiment with inoculations against smallpox during the Qing dynasty. These primitive methods smeared the stuff of smallpox lesions or scabs directly into the nasal mucosa either by a wet smear or dry powder. Yet this still allowed the inactivated infectious agent to enter via the nasal mucosa and activate the proper Tai Yang reaction.

Vaccinations provoke an immune response that causes our B cells (from the bone marrow) to produce antibodies and display antigens to which our immune cells then recognize and respond. When the pathogen is injected directly into the bloodstream instead of its usual entrance via the mucous membranes, however, it can produce Heat and inflammation at the Blood level, potentially overwhelming the immune system and causing latency.

To further complicate matters, the newer DNA and mRNA vaccinations bypass the usual routes of entrance entirely. Contrary to the progression from Wei Qi to Yin Qi to Yuan Qi, these vaccines go directly to the Yuan Qi to alter the Constitutional level, especially Chong and Wei Mai. While these pharmaceutical agents are very new and still considered experimental, at present we know that they can result in myriad potential immunologic and reproductive alterations, immune suppression, recurring infections, wheezing, allergic reactions, sleep apnea, exacerbations of autoimmune tendencies, and increased blood clotting, and they alter the relationship of angiotensin I (which becomes deficient) and angiotensin II (which becomes overactive), resulting in blood pressure spikes. They impact how the Yuan Qi interacts with both the Ying and Wei Qi, modifying Kidney Jing, suppressing Wei Qi, and causing Liver Yang rising and Phlegm and Blood stasis. In 2021, Covid-19 vaccine sales catapulted Pfizer to the number one drug sales position in the world, generating 36.9 billion dollars with their Comirnaty vaccine, while Moderna's Spikevax came in third at $17.7 billion (Dunleavy, 2022). When drug sales began to decline, boosters were developed to prevent further slumps. Pfizer still held the lead in 2022, as Comirnaty sales reached $55.9 billion. Paxlovid by Pfizer came in fourth and Spikevax by Moderna fell to fifth, each bringing in over $18 billion. We will likely witness many more long-term sequelae from these new pharmacological bad boys over time. (Conveniently, over ten of the top 50 best-selling pharmaceuticals in 2022 address autoimmune presentations caused by breaches in the Wei Qi.)

Adjuvants like aluminum are added to some vaccines to enhance the recipient's response to the vaccine. Aluminum, which is a neurotoxin, can remain in the body and settle in the tissues, making it difficult to detoxify, meanwhile producing Heat, Fire Toxins, and Stasis.

All vaccinations, whether they disrupt the Blood or Yuan level first, violate the Yuan Qi in order to stimulate an immediate Wei Qi reaction, a Yang effect, although the immune system often won't even mount a response to heat-treated inactive viruses. The reaction to the vaccine depends in a large part on the strength of the Yuan Qi. In response to the surge of Yang Qi, the body may have to utilize some Yin fluid, Jing, Jin/Ye, or Blood to attempt to hold latent any resultant Toxic Heat, which may result in an increase in clotting factors. Ongoing divergent treatments may also be used to treat latent autoimmune reactions, and the Luo vessels can clear Heat at the organ level. Pc 6 and Ht 5 are very useful for patients who experience post-vaccine Heart symptoms.

Bacterial invasions can be secondary respiratory infections subsequent to viral infections. They can also enter the body via the urinary tract or the digestive system; they can also gain entrance directly into the bloodstream through a breach in the skin. Bacterial pathogens are both Hot and somewhat Damp (this is what makes them linger), and are mainly drawn to the Fu organs. The Fu organs are naturally predisposed to bacteria through the gut's microflora. The secondary Yang Ming level (St/Ll) wages the response to these Heat pathogens with its abundant Qi and Blood. Bacteria often come on board secondary to a viral infection while the immune system is busy or overwhelmed as Heat increases and hangs around.

Antibiotics

- Aminoglycosides: amikacin (Amikin), gentamicin (Garamycin), kan-amycin (Kantrex), neomycin (Neo-Fradin), netilmicin (Netromycin), tobramycin (Nebcin), paramomycin (Humatin), streptomycin, spectin-omycin (Trobicin)

- Ansamycin: rifaximin (Xifaxan)
- Carbapenems: ertapenem (Invent), doripenem (Doribax), imepenem/cilastatin (Primaxin), meropenem (Merrem)
- First-generation cephalosporins: cefadroxil (Duricef), cefazolin (Ancef, Kefzol), cephradine, cephapirin, cephalothin, cefalexin (Keflex)
- Second-generation cephalosporins: cefaclor (Distaclor, Ceclor, Rancor), cefoxitin, cefotetan (Cefotan), cefamandole, cefmetazole, cefonicid, loracarbef, cefprozil (Cefzil), cefuroxime (Ceftin, Zinacef)
- Third-generation cephalosporins: cefixime (Cefspan, Suprax), cefdinir (Omnicef, Cefdiel), cefditoren (Sectracef, Meiact), cefotaxine (Claforan), cefpodoxime (Vantin, Banadoz), ceftazidime (Fortaz, Ceptaz), ceftibuten (Cedax), ceftizoxime, moxalactam, ceftriaxone (Rocephin)
- Fourth-generation cephalosporins: cefepime (Maxipime)
- Fifth-generation cephalosporins: ceftaroline fossil (Teflaro), ceftobiprole (Zeftera)
- Glycopeptides: teicoplanin (Targocid), vancomycin (Vancocin), telavancin (Vibativ), dalbavancin (Dalvance), oritavancin (Orbactiv)
- Lincosamides: clindamycin (Cleocin), lincomycin (Lincocin)
- Lipopeptide: daptomycin (Cybicin)
- Macrolides: azithromycin (Zithromax, Somme, Xithrone), clarithyromycin (Biaxin), erythromycin (Erythrocin, Erythroped), roxithromycin, telithromycin (Setek), spiramycin (Rovamycine), fidaxomicin (Dificid), aztreonam (Azactam)
- Nitrofurans: furazolidone (Furoxone), nitrofurantoin (Macrodantin, Macrobid)
- Oxazolidinones: linezoid (Zyvox), posizolid, radezolid, torezolid (Sivextro)
- Penicillins: amoxocillin (Novamox, Amoxil), ampicillin, aziocillin, dicloxacillin, flucloxacillin, mezlocillin, methicillin, nafcillin, oxacillin, penicillin G (Pfizerpen), penicillin V, piperacillin, temocillin, ticarcillin
- Penicillin combinations: amoxicillin/clavulanate (Augmentin), ampicillin/dulbactam (Unasyn), piperacillin/tazobactam (Zosyn), ticarcillin/clavulanate (Timentin)
- Polypeptides: bacitracin, colistin (Coly-Mycin-S), polymyxin B
- Quinolones/Fluoroquinolones: ciproflaxacin (Cipro, Ciproxin,

Ciprobay), enoxacin (Penetrex), gatifloxacin (Tequin), gemifloxacin (Factive), levoflaxacin (Levaquin), lornefloxacin (Maxaquin), moxifloxacin (Avelox), nadifloxacin, nalidixic acid (NegGram), norfloxacin (Noroxin), ofloaxacin (Ocuflox)

- Sulfonamides: mafenide (Sulfamylon), sulfacetamide (Sulamyd, Bleph-10), sulfadiazine (Micro-Sulfon), silver sulfadiazine (Silvadine), sulfamethizole (Thiosulfil Forte), sulfadimethoxine (Di-Methox, Albon), sulfamethoxazole (Gentanol), sulfanilamide, sulfasalazine (Azulfidine), sulfisoxazole (Gentrisin), trimethoprim-sulfamethoxazole (Bactrim, Septra), sulfonamidochrysoidine (Prontosil)
- Tetracyclines: used for chlamydia, syphilis, Lyme disease, mycoplasma, acne, malaria: demeclocycline (Declomycin), doxycycline (Vibramycin), metacycline, minocycline (Mirocin), oxytetracycline (Terramycin), tetracycline (Sumycin, Achromycin V, Steclin)
- Others: arsphenamine (Salvarsan), chloramphenicol (Chloromycetin), fosfomycin (Monaural), fusidic acid (Fucidin), metronidazole (Flagyl), mupirocin (Bactroban), platensimycin, quinupristin/dalfopristin (Synercid), thiamphenicol, tigecycline (Tigacyl), tinidazole (Tindamax, Fasigyn), trimethoprim (Proloprim, Trimpex)

Prior to 1936, 30 percent of all deaths were due to bacterial infections. The development of antibiotics revolutionized health care, but as most medical advances prove over time, we aren't smarter than nature. As science developed more sophisticated and intricate instrumentation to peer into the stuff of atoms, neutrinos and quarks appeared. Similarly, as medicine has been able to identify more and more bacterial agents and develop specific antibiotics to target them, bacterial pathogens have become smarter and have cleverly morphed into new antibiotic-resistant strains. Antibiotics have become so common, many people expect a prescription whenever they become sick, even with viruses, on which they have no effect whatever. Pediatricians often prescribe antibiotics not because the child needs them, but so the parents feel that at least something is being done for their sick baby. Inappropriate antibiotic prescriptions might be the easiest way to move patients in and out of the clinic. According to a study on the appropriateness of outpatient antibiotic in BMJ 2019, 364, out of over 27 million patients and 15 million antibiotic prescriptions, only 12.8 percent were considered appropriate. 35.5 percent were potentially appropriate, 23.2 percent were inappropriate, and 28.5 percent were not associated with a recent diagnostic code. This is significant in the development of antibiotic resistant strains. Fortunately, we can help address the underlying predisposition to recurrent bacterial infections.

Bacterial disease mechanisms include External Wind, Dampness, and Heat. Pattern discrimination may also involve Heat toxins, Qi vacuity, Yin vacuity, or lingering Damp Heat. To avoid the need for antibiotics and reduce bacterial resistance, many bacterial infections can be resolved by clearing Yang Ming Heat (Ll 11) and resolving Dampness (Sp 9) while reinforcing the immune system (Ren 6, St 36, UB 20, UB 21, UB 23). Herbs that clear both Dampness and Heat like Huang Lian, Huang Bai, and Huang Qin, among others, have antibacterial properties, while Huang Qi strengthens the Lung and Spleen Qi by encouraging production of immature immune cells in the bone marrow and activation in the lymph tissues. Raw Huang Qi also invigorates cilia in the mucosal tissues.

Needless to say, antibiotics don't kill viruses. They specifically destroy bacteria by attacking their cell walls (Wei Qi), interfering with their ability to reproduce, or their ability to make the necessary proteins needed to survive (Yang effects). We can categorize all of these mechanisms as Heat, which antibiotics Cool. Usually, bacterial overgrowth initially responds well to specific antibiotics. Being Cold in nature, antibiotics clear Heat, but the Cold often injures the Spleen and worsens Dampness, often causing some bacteria to remain and proliferate in the now Damp environment. This is also why yeast overgrowth is common after antibiotic administration.

Antibacterial side effects include nausea, vomiting, diarrhea, abdominal pain, rashes, dizziness, seizures, allergic and anaphylactic reactions, and potential organ damage. Each also carries specific risks; for example, penicillins can cause deadly allergic reactions, jaundice, and urinary difficulty. Antibiotics with sulfur, like Bactrim, have more of a warming effect. Tetracyclines can cause serum sickness, hypertension, sun sensitivity, and tooth discoloration. Macrolides (Azithromyacin) cause more Dampening signs like diminishing taste and vaginal discharge. Cephalosporins (Keflex) can cause joint pain and damage the Kidneys; fluoroquinolones (Cipro) can cause fainting, hallucinations, and liver injury. They are very cooling, and long-term use can bind to minerals in the bones, leading to osteoporosis. Glycopeptides (Vancomycin) can induce mood changes and cause low back pain as well as induce anaphylactic reactions. Antibiotics often induce latency and do not provide a route for detoxification. Thus, the condition may lie dormant, and when the Qi, Blood, or body fluids diminish, we may have to deal with their effects when more serious diseases present later on. Tai Yang conditions are usually treated with spicy and warm herbs to expel the Wind. Antibiotics have the opposite effects, and can push the pathogen further in.

If someone is taking antibiotics, we won't necessarily be prescribing Tai Yang formulas, but formulas that prevent progression to other stages, like Bai Hu Tang for Yang Ming, and Xiao Chai Hu Tang for Shao Yang. For patients who have been on prolonged antibiotics, our treatment principles will need to include resolving residual Dampness and Cold, while fortifying the Spleen, recommending prebiotics, and encouraging the bowels to move.

If a Tai Yang condition has been treated with antibiotics, look out for Dampness and Cold. Unresolved Cold Dampness can drain downward and develop into cystitis, for which Cipro is often prescribed. While they are on the antibiotics, we can prescribe something like Wu Ling San to prevent the Dampness from spreading while they continue taking them. Replace Bai Zhu with Cang Zhu, which is warming and has antifungal properties, as there is still a possibility for a viral flare up, or the development of fungal infections.

Antibiotics destroy gut bacteria, which Ll 4 and St 42 can address. Recent studies have shown that even one course of antibiotics can upset the gut bacteria, especially bifidobacterium, for up to two years. Supplementing with probiotics, especially bifidus, can also help restore damaged gut bacteria. Geng Mi, non-glutinous rice, can help engender fluids, as well as soups from fermented soy beans or Dan Dou Chi. Since antibiotics impact the absorption of B12 and folic acid, the immune system may be further compromised.

Antiparasitics

Helminths are worm-like parasites including flukes, roundworms, and tape-worms that can survive and thrive living off of their human hosts. They are obtained through contaminated food, water, or certain insect bites. They can live in the intestinal tract for years without becoming symptomatic, but often cause intestinal symptoms, fatigue, fever, weight loss, skin rashes, and neuro-logical symptoms. They can also hide out in nutrient-rich environments like the gallbladder. Gallbladder cleanses often purge gall stones and parasites.

Chinese medicine has an entire school of attacking and purging, which is one of our approaches to expelling parasites. Wu Mei Wan is a classical formula that warms the viscera while clearing Heat, coursing the Liver, recti-fying the Qi, harmonizing the Stomach, and expelling worms by moving them downward. Worms are Yin pathogens, and when we alter the environment parasites thrive in, they will tend to vacate the premises. Wormwood and black walnut husk are antiparasitic, as is clove oil, which can also destroy their eggs. Diatomaceous earth can cut into the outer coating of parasites, dehydrating them. Eating a diet devoid of sugar, grain, and processed foods, while including garlic, onions, and scallions, can produce a more Yang envi-ronment which is less hospitable to parasites.

Antihelminthics are a group of antiparasitic drugs that expel worms:

- Albendazole (Albenza)
- Mendazole (Emverm, Vermox)
- Pyrantel (Ascarel)
- Ivermectin (Stromectol)
- Triclabendazole (Egaten)
- Miltefosine (Impavido)

Antihelminthics are selectively toxic to parasites, targeting vital metabolic processes primarily in the parasite and to a lesser degree in its mammalian host. Albendazole, for example, binds to tubulin, the protein fibers that constitute microtubules which serve as a skeletal system for living cells in parasitic worms. Avermectin, which originated from a microorganism found in Japanese soil, was discovered in the late 1970s. Its derivative, ivermectin, which blocks glutamate and gamma-aminobutyric acid (GABA) and glu-tamine-gated chloride channels, has been found effective against parasites, scabies, ticks, lice, bacteria, viruses, and many other infestations in mammals. Antihelminthic agents aim to paralyze or starve the parasites, after which they are expelled. These drugs may become toxic to the host as well, however, and can induce serious side effects, including stomach pain, nausea, vomiting, diarrhea, headaches, dizziness, fever, chills, rashes, body aches, joint pain, and tender lymph nodes. They incite Yang reactivity by heightening our own immunologic reactions, while in heavy doses over time these drugs will become toxic to the Spleen and Liver.

Fungal infections are drawn to Damp, and like the naturally fluid-filled Curious Organs: the uterus, genitals, joints, bones, brain, and gallbladder. While it is common to encounter vaginal yeast infections in female populations, candida can also proliferate in the prostate gland in men, where it can fester for years. Sugar intensifies Dampness and moldy overgrowth, which is why after eating sweet or fermented foods, fungal infections are often aggravated. Damp and humid environments encourage fungal overgrowth, and the body has difficulty drying the fluids on its own. Fermented Damp environments become acidic. Draining Dampness or invigorating the Spleen to resolve Dampness may help, but often we need to resolve mucus and Phlegm from protein break down; get into the Shao Yang (GB/SJ) level to scour the Damp pathogens from the Gallbladder; as well as utilize San Jiao to restore clear waterways. Fungal infections can linger in the Damp terrain, and during times of immune system stress can gain entrance into the marrow to cause neurotoxicity.

Eating a more alkaline diet will help resolve the conditions that lead to fungal overgrowth, eliminating breads, yeast, dairy, sugar, fruit, and fermented foods and beverages. Mushrooms are fungi that grow in damp environments; they are governed by Water, absorb heavy metal toxins and pollutants, and help the body drain Dampness and rid Phlegm stasis. Interestingly, reishi and chaga have antifungal effects on the candida albicans biofilm. Aspirin comes from the bark of a willow tree that grows in swampy environments, which provides its antifungal effects. Our treatments must focus on (aromatically) drying Dampness and Phlegm, clearing Heat, and we may need to tonify underlying Qi or Yang deficiency.

Antifungals

- Polyenes: amphotericin B, candicin, filipin, hamycin, natamycin, nystatin, rimocidin

- Azoles:
    - Imidazoles: bifonazole, butoconazole, clotrimazole, econazole, fenticonazole, isoconazole, ketoconazole, luliconazole, miconazole, omoconazzole, oxiconazole, sertaconazole, sulconazole, tioconazole
    - Triazoles: albaconazole, efinaconazole, epoxiconazole, fluconazole, isavuconazole, itraconazole, posaconazole, propiconazole, ravuconazole, terconazole, voriconazole
    - Thiazoles: abafungin
    - Allyamines: butenafine, naftifine, terbinafine
    - Echinocandins: anidulafungin, caspofungin, micafungin
    - Triterpenoids: ibrexafungerp
- Others: acrisorcin, amorolfine, auroras, benzoic acid, carbon fuchsin, chlorophetanol, ciclopirox, clioquinol, coal tar, copper sulfate, diiodohydroxyquinoline (Iodoquinol), flucytosine (5-fluorocytosine), fumagilin, griseofulvin, miltefosine, nikkomucin, orotomide, piroctone olamine, pentanenitrile, potassium iodide, potassium permanganate, selenium disulfide, sodium thiosulfate, sulfur, toinaftawte, triacetin, undecylenic acid, zinc pyrithione

Antifungals, also known as antimycotics, are medications that can treat fungal infections like ringworm, athlete's foot, dandruff, vaginal yeast infections, nail fungus, thrush and systemic infiltrations like aspergillosis, and candidemia, a fungal infection of the blood. They target fungal cell walls and membranes to either kill the fungal cells or prevent them from proliferating. The most common antimycotics are azoles, which interfere with an enzyme necessary for the cell wall. They are categorized either as imidazoles (like ketoconazole) or triazoles (like fluconazole). Polyenes like nystatin and amphotericin B make the cell walls more porous, so their contents can burst. The Chinese herbal formula Cao Huang Gui Xiang (Gan Cao, Da Huang, Rou Gui, Guang Huo Xiang), effective at resolving candida albicans, also inhibits biofilm and filament formation. Oils from oregano, clove, and mint, among others, also have antifungal properties.

Because fungi are very proliferative and linger in Damp environments, antifungals are often prescribed for months at a time. Unfortunately, because of their toxicity, they also are known to cause liver damage, and they interact negatively with many other medications. In order to terminate these Damp pathogens, antimycotics must have properties that penetrate Dampness. Their effects don't tend to cause Dryness as we might expect, however, but more Heat signs. Side effects include acid reflux, stomach pain, nausea, diarrhea, constipation, dizziness, and severe fatigue, as well as itchy, burning skin and rashes. Other rarer side effects include urine changes, muscle pains and cramps, hair loss, bleeding, bruising, allergic reactions, mood changes, paranoia, and hallucinations. The mechanisms antifungals employ to penetrate the Dampness and Phlegm result in counterflow Qi, and Toxic Heat reactions.

CHAPTER 4

Drugs That Affect the Mind

There is a journey you must take.
It is a journey without destination.
There is no map.
Your soul will lead you.
And you can take nothing with you.

—Meister Eckhart

Shen

The living of our lives brings us closer to or further away from the awareness of the Way and its healing power within us. The *Nei Jing* tells us that all diseases are rooted in Shen, and the Heart is the only true healer. When we are ill at ease, there is always something wrong with our perception of reality. The Shen, like undifferentiated light, extends the subtle and miraculous influences from beyond to shine on and through our life. The Shen are home to the Heart, providing conscious awareness, the ability to feel, sense, and experience life through a personal lens. When the Shen are clear, there is a glow to our complexion and a brightness to our eyes, as if they are backlit. If our personal experience of life is darkened, the facial light often becomes somewhat dulled.

The Shen, as emissaries from Heaven, are able to resolve all states of dis-ease as they focus the healing power and wisdom of the eternal within us, shining away all states of mental dullness from their home in the Heart.

Remember, the Blood follows the Qi, and the Qi follows the Xin. As Big (cosmic) Shen manifests as small (personal) Shen, it brings with it a mandate from Heaven which defines how the major events in our life unfold, including the emotional challenges which can be the underlying cause of disease, especially if we try to avoid the opportunities they provide. The *Ling Shu* stresses the importance of attending to the spirit first, so it can manifest the three qualities of Shen:

- Harmonized Qi and Blood.
- Clear communication between Ying and Wei Qi.
- The Zang Fu are complete, and have come to express the highest virtues of each element.

When any of these three qualities are deranged, Shen disturbances may result. There are four cardinal signs of a disruption in spirit (when the mind function of small Shen is disordered). Shen themselves are not altered, but our mind's ability to relate to them can become confused. Shen disturbances may then manifest as any of these four symptomatic expressions:

- Fatigue—or just being tired of life.
- Forgetfulness—where life loses its meaning.
- Uncertainty—having no direction in life.
- Insomnia—a restless, preoccupied mind that can't relax.

True healing is not the mere resolution of symptoms, but a deep understanding of and respect for their causes. And often the causes of Shen disturbances arise from much deeper realms than the tips of the psychic icebergs of which we are aware. We all experience our own personal psycho-emotional interpretations of life. Yet underneath them all lies the greatest unitive state of unconditional peace, as well as the greatest form of suffering in human life—a feeling of being lost and alone, separate from our source and all of creation. Unfortunately, this is what many of us experience in our darkest hours, and what most of us spend our lives attempting to avoid, escape, or overcome. Yet, if we can get through the barrier of our own projected phantoms, the inner realms invite us to experience the source of life as our very self, without division. This earthly journey leads us through peaks and valleys, highs and lows, and we are meant to experience them all, until we are shed of every attachment that stands between us and Heaven and we find our way home to the profundity of who we really are.

Many, if not most, human beings in our society are addicted to the egoic thought system predicated on the belief that we should avoid all pain and discomfort and desire only pleasure and comfort. It is this dynamic which causes suffering, because life involves both pleasure and pain. The wisdom tradition of our forebears viewed life as a journey where we begin all essence and, if we follow our destiny, we end up all spirit. If we honor this view, we see that three overarching themes guide us from one phase to another as we redeem Shen from Jing.

The first phase is one of survival, where we care for our bodily identity and protect our physicality. The second phase is governed by our social inter-actions that form our psycho-emotional, relational identity. The third and final phase is one of differentiation, where we come to see who we really are, and sometimes more importantly, who we are not. Discernment provides directionality to the Hun so our cosmic identity can reveal our true nature. Although we incorporate all three levels within us, as we transition from one dominant phase to another, we are invited to give up our previous identities and the worldviews they held. And the price for these alchemical transmu-tations requires us to enter into periods of darkness, where we can't see the light. Call it the dark night of the soul, or the eye of the needle, there is one thing for sure—the alchemical cauldron is rarely perfumed, cushioned, or decorated with niceties. It's meant to be empty and devoid of our attachments so we can enter the liminal space between worlds where there's nothing but us and our creator; not as two. Spiritual growth may hurt as we shed the skins of our previous selves, and all that upheld them. But we all were prepared for this in-utero. During the ninth lunar month of pregnancy, the light of mother's Shen is withdrawn from the fetus. This causes it to rotate and turn downward, to look for another source of light that can only be found by passing into the lower Yin. We were made to be rebirthed through our pain, not to try to escape from it.

The 13th-century Sufi poet Rumi's poetry abounds with instructions like: *The hurt we embrace becomes joy*; and from *The Guest House*, that even *depression* and *meanness*, as well as *dark thoughts, shame and malice*, should be gratefully welcomed and invited in. The founders of Alcoholics Anonymous, who seemed to have the corner on psychic suffering, found comfort in recognizing that *pain is the touchstone of all spiritual progress*, a quote likely borrowed from the fifth century Greek Aeschylus: *He who learns must suffer. And even in our sleep, pain that cannot forget falls drop by drop upon the heat, and in our own despair and against our will, comes wisdom to us by the awful grace of God.* The Buddha said that *desire leads to suffering,* Jesus said *resist ye not evil,* and another biblical character who was no stranger to pain said that suffering produces perseverance; perseverance, character; and character, hope. True hope does not merely project itself out as an idea of a better improved future, for that reeks of expectation, which belongs to the Liver. We are saturated by expectation, a form of resistance that demands things be better or at least different than they are. True hope, on the other hand, resides in the present moment as a buoyancy of Heart, where full acceptance allows a pause from past conditioning that spurs us on, no matter the circumstances. And those who have come to know this state say it is precisely because of the psychic suffering they have endured and come through that their Hearts have opened to an unconditional way of being in the world. I'm pretty sure nobody ever said they awakened by medicating their pain. We simply cannot overcome the ego's suffering by trying to make it feel better.

The *Tao te Ching* reinforces, verse after verse, that humanity shouldn't try to force harmony; the whole adjusts by itself, whether we are speaking of the macrocosm or the microcosm. The Tao doesn't take sides; it gives birth to both good and evil, pleasure and pain. The Way is a pathless path into the vast unknown depths of life, the only place where we can find and live the destiny Heaven inscribed into our very beings. And if we pay attention to the truth within, anything less tends to cause mental disturbance. And mental disturbance, if heeded as part of the path, leads us back to the truth within. Whenever we are upset, for any reason, we are in a state of resistance, which dams up the flow of what is. It isn't until we face what is, including our response to whatever might be upsetting us, that we can find where our own inner conflict resides. If we only mute our pain, we will never find our way to transcend it and enter the full expanse of our authentic personhood, both innocent and wise.

When we come to know the limitless expanse of our Heart-Mind, it is understood that all illness is mental illness, and that medicine and psychology are one thing, for as we know the Qi follows the Mind. We are meant to have a still mind, rooted in a quiet Heart. The natural condition is to be immersed in this serene and constant state. Spirits inhabit the void of the Heart, allowing us to know ourselves through a constant flowing stream of consciousness that leads us toward the peace and joy of self-awareness. But we are advised not to force stillness of mind or escape the world in order to achieve tranquility, for that is just resistance that bypasses the curriculum we came to learn.

The Shen also include the Hun and the Po souls. The seven Po give rise to our most challenging life issues. They are our greatest teachers; until we have learned their lessons, they remain in the deep shadows of our internal landscape, waiting to be activated so they can help us progress.

Programmed by Heaven at conception, they lie like dormant serpents in the underbelly, and when it is time for our lessons to emerge, predetermined life challenges will change the internal environment and wake up the Po which, if resisted, can fester, anguishing body, mind, and soul. We can't speed them along, slow them down, jump over or sidestep them. While we may try numerous ways to escape, medicate, or distract ourselves from them, they will re-emerge, often with a vengeance. Yet when we begin to recognize them, we can bow down to them as the benevolent guiding spirits that they are. We simply cannot avoid our conflicts if we are to overcome them. The way of mastery is to be with our own hauntings, *Gui* 鬼, so they don't become *Mo* 魔, evil spirits; they instead transform into benevolent allies which teach us we have nothing to fear.

The seven Po deities (Yin, Yang, Shen, Qi, Jing, Longevity, and Sex) create the necessary friction for us to overcome on our life path. These clever little energetic phantoms take the pure light of Shen and make consciousness believe that shadows have power. Seen as the animal souls, they are governed by the moon, and could correspond with the seven emotional extremes, seven deadly sins, or the seven temptations. In the body-mind, these egoic powers consist of distortions like darkness, overemphasis on the body, excess desires, clinging attachment, ignorance, forgetting, anger, and rage—extreme forms of resistance. But they are unique for each of us.

While the classics depicted them as ghoulish figures with names like Thief Swallower and Dead Dog, the powers of Yin usually get a bad rap. While they are not to be blindly indulged, they are not "bad," nor are they to be avoided; they bring to life the most challenging issues which can force us out of a mundane ego-based existence to a sacred life in service to the whole. They provide the alchemical fuel that propels us all the way from the underworld to heaven's gates, deep within our own psyche. These inner hauntings have a long history of being disowned, projected outwards, and called evil spirits. Yet when we can turn the light of consciousness around and meet them with understanding, our most demonic emotional issues may become our greatest assets. When we go directly through the eye of the needle of our own fears, they are literally transformed into the wisdom of the lesson learned. Our constitution is cleansed.

The Po souls give rise to our baser instincts, including the desire for food, sex, and material wealth. Like hungry ghosts in their extreme forms, addictions and substance abuse belong to the Po realm. Those who need to control their intake are precisely the ones who cannot. Likewise, those who need most to undo negative or traumatic messages from their past simply cannot reach them through conscious effort, conventional psychotherapy, or pharmaceutical distortion. While changing negative thoughts to more positive ones might help that over which the conscious mind has control, we cannot control the unconscious. As these egoic powers that make the body seem more real than the spirit come out of hiding, we have to look at them and confront the ways we have been under their spell, albeit unknowingly. And for this we must be willing to turn toward our most challenging issues. And in order to see clearly in the dark, we need to bring the light of consciousness with us. That light is offered by the Hun.

The three Hun, in communication with both Heaven and the seven Po, help mediate our place between individualized Shen and cosmic Shen. They provide the intangible aspects of our higher functions: one carries the fetal spark of light; one determines the things toward which we will be attracted; and one the light of our intellect. In order to accurately utilize the Hun, they must interact with the Po. As we dare to enter into our inner darkness, the light can shine within, and the Hun achieve greater, more expansive vision. A common mistake humans have made for far too long is to reject their baser instincts or suppress their most glaring issues, and "choose" the light over the darkness. This preference for Yang has made us an imbalanced, Yin-deficient species. The Hun and Po souls separate, keeping the subconscious in the dark, where much of humanity remains blind to their own inner work and lives, according to Zhuang Zi, as walking corpses, recirculating the same putrid issues in their lives over and over. In Chapter 8, the *Ling Shu* describes a condition where the Hun and Po become injured, making us crazy. Because the Po's gravitational pull is in and down toward that which is unconscious, the conscious Hun must move within to interact with them so the light of wisdom can help us navigate in the dark, where our most powerful lessons are learned. While this process may feel maddening at times, the Po are great allies whom we are meant to meet and befriend. As we shine the light within, eventually the Hun rise and the Po exit. By following the Way, we can become like the immortals, who danced with their own darkness, trading their egos to embody the light of Shen Ming. Deeply rooted in Yin, darkness within darkness, they remain eternal beacons lighting the Way, never afraid of the dark.

The Po are intimately related to the Kidney energies and Jing. Conflicts in the Jing deplete and corrode this precious resource. But if we shine the light of Shen into the dark potential of Jing, we begin to know and live our purpose. Li Shi Zhen said, *If we can preserve Jing, the Shen will be bright. If Shen is bright, there will be long life.* When we resist the invitations offered by the shadowy realm to examine and awaken from our fears, our consciousness remains unable to penetrate into the place where the virtue of wisdom is given. As such, we haven't become a very wise species. We keep trying to get away from our ghoulish little friends who can actually wake us up from some rather insane societal agreements. While mind- and mood-altering substances can make us feel better, they keep us small, contained, and generally more content with the status quo. Whether we use food, alcohol, or drugs, those with antidepressant effects temporarily mute or lift us out of our shadows, keeping them safely hidden underground. Until, of course, they stop working. And anxiolytics keep us blanketed from the awareness of the gifts our deepest hauntings can reveal. As Lao Tau said, knowing yourself is true wisdom, and mastering yourself is true power. This type of power simply embarrasses the medical establishment.

The master concerns himself with the depths
Rather than the surface

—*Tao te Ching, Chapter 38*

During one retreat I worked with an acupuncturist/yoga instructor who defined herself as "light and love," and claimed she had no anger, although she often became depressed because of the hatred she saw "in the world." She had been on Xiao Yao San for years, and was quite adept at masking her negative states. She dressed in flowing clothes, and it seemed that there was quite a bit of effort to present herself in a spiritual, healing posture. While her superficial appearance was all smiles and bliss, her clenched teeth and red neck and ears betrayed the anger she was denying in herself and projecting outward. Her eyes weren't lacking Shen; the lights were on, but there wasn't much presence to them. There was also a sadness about her. Her pulse was very wiry on the surface and empty underneath. I poked at her demeanor a few times until her mask began to crack, and the truth came out. She was flaming mad, and equally horrified to admit it. She had grown up in a home with a rageful father, and swore she would never become an angry adult, making her unable to acknowledge her true feelings. Ongoing treatment included helping her through the fury she was desperately trying to avoid acknowledging, harmonizing the Liver, and working with the second trajectory of the Chong Mai, needling Ki 24, which was especially reactive. Beneath her resistance she carried an ever-present sorrow, which Ki 26 and Lu 3 then helped integrate. She then found an even deeper light—the one her grief revealed—which gave her access to a deeper and more profound healing power. Now that she no longer had to fix herself into a mold of what she thought being "spiritual" looked like, she was able to offer this gift to others plagued with anger, resistance, and grief.

When we adhere too closely to what society deems "normal" or "good," we conform to an external pattern which may not be all that sane in the first place, or certainly might go against our own inner truth. Hence, when the Tao is lost, we resort to ideas of what is virtuous or moral and thus begins the deterioration process. We have to learn to speak from our internal truth rather than medicating our discomfort, otherwise we may never learn the lessons we are here to accomplish.

Early in life, emotional stimuli meet our constitutional and temperamental tendencies, generating insidious and hidden emotional patterns that produce bioelectrical charges in the nervous system, affecting our circulatory rhythms, breathing patterns, hormonal and digestive functions, and immune defenses. When these disruptions are identified with, or are taken to be our very selves, we are no longer in possession of ourselves. We lose our natural state and instead become possessed by emotional states, to which we are often blind. Because our senses draw us outward, we tend to remain unaware of this internal tension. In *When the Body Says No*, Gabor Maté (2011) states that when emotions are repressed, this inhibition disarms the body's defenses against illness. Our upright Qi can no longer stand up against evil Qi. When our internal rhythms no longer sync with the flow of life, we lose harmony with nature, and no longer experience ease. Our neurobiology follows.

As the orifices of the Heart become clouded, Fire loses its clear connection with Kidney Water, which ceases to nourish Liver Blood. The unanchored Liver ascends, loses charge of the Hun, the sinews stiffen, and movements become erratic as Fire flares upward. When the Spleen weakens, anxiety, worry, and preoccupation fester and injure the spirits which are trapped by the Spleen's obsessive tendencies. The Lungs can no longer descend or direct the Qi. The officials disassociate from one another, the Heart and Shen no longer have a place on which to rely; thought becomes scattered, connections and mastery are lost. There is no basis for clear thinking or reflection. The spirits become agitated in this environment and take flight; no longer present in the Heart, one loses the ability to know or be oneself. When the spirits are no longer able to express themselves, the vitality of Ming Men is disturbed. Cold can enter and freeze the Heart, and lock up the diaphragm, producing a feeling of malaise. When we no longer know who we truly are, ailments galore may arise. Eczema, back pain, infertility, and cancer are some of the innumerable physical manifestations. Depending on our temperament, blame, victimization, shame, and guilt are a few of its mental projections. Beneath the branch symptoms, though, we find the root: we have lost possession of ourselves, and harmony with the Way.

And the only way to find our way again is to start with the out-picturings and trace our way back to the source. If we dare to pay attention, we often find that our symptoms are but the thread that we can follow on our return trip home. The reclamation of ourselves is no small feat.

The Blood follows the Qi
The Qi follows the Heart-Mind
The Mind follows the Shen
The Shen follows the Tao
The Tao follows Itself

The Qi follows the Heart-Mind, and the Shen is most present in that which requires our full attention in the moment. Wei Qi is responsible for our moods; Ying Qi and Blood for our emotional makeup; and Yuan Qi for our constitutional tendencies. Depressed states can originate from and permeate all three levels. Our source connects us most deeply to each other through the One Mind. Most issues of anxiety and depression arise from feeling separate and alone, disconnected from our origin, cut off from parts of ourselves and others. Wei Qi connects us superficially to other bodies and external factors, which may then trigger internal responses, but external circumstances don't cause depression. The outside world is a projection of our internal state. We see not what is, but what we are. The Ying Qi and Blood levels provide our thought life and emotional landscape. When our conditioned illusions defile the clarity of a pure Heart and cloud its orifices, the illuminating inner light that we are vibrates at a lower pitch, the windows of Heaven darken, and we begin to lose our way. We close off our Hearts and begin to feel separate and alone. The result—depressed moods, repressed emotions, imbalanced neurotransmitters, and misfiring of the nervous system.

Neurotransmitters

Neurotransmitters are small signaling molecules, originating from Kidney Yin, Yang, and Jing, that neurons secrete across a synapse to affect other cells. Together with neuropeptides, larger proteins associated with the Blood that are found all over the neuron, these chemical messengers transmit our feeling states. Since no major drug classes have yet been developed that can selectively modify neuropeptides, pharmaceutical companies have focused on developing drugs that manipulate neurotransmitters. As neurotransmitters are released by the neuron, they are recycled by the synapse through a process called reuptake, which regulates the level of neurotransmitters and the duration of their signals.

We each carry an internal chemical pharmacy whose constituents are activated by the energies, often unconscious, that make us feel elated, sorrowful, or terrified as the Qi follows the Heart-Mind. We are meant to honor the full array of feeling states, but not become swept away by them such that we lose hold of the Heart center. There's a lot that we can learn about ourselves and our relationship with the world when we understand their movements. Certain neurotransmitters like norepinephrine are stimulatory and have a Yang effect; others like GABA inhibit central nervous system excitatory messages to regulate sleep and waking cycles. When deficient, anxiety results, and when in excess, disordered sleeping and eating patterns may develop. Dopamine, which is involved in smooth movement, pleasure, attention, and learning, inhibits excitatory messages and keeps Yang in check. Its functions might be likened to Liver Blood engendering Heart Qi.

Serotonin is an inhibitory neurotransmitter that regulates many physiologic processes and mood states. Derived from L-Tryptophan, this regulatory pineal hormone is produced in response to daylight exposure. Serotonin is increased by exercise, stimulating activities, and being outdoors. This Yang action draws us up and out, gives a sense of confidence, and inhibits the downward Yin movement that may be associated with depressed moods. When exposed to dark, serotonin is converted to its Yin expression, melatonin, to help us tune inward and sleep. Like the Qiao Mai, serotonin and melatonin regulate light and dark signals, our ability to go within and find comfort, and to look outward and find new possibilities. Norepinephrine is a Yang-invigorating neurotransmitter released by the adrenal glands in response to stressors in order to increase heart rate and raise blood pressure to mobilize the brain, large muscle groups, and eyes to act strongly and quickly to escape from danger. And orexin is a Yang neurotransmitter in the brain that affects mood and cognition, keeping us awake, aroused, and hungry.

But lest you think neurotransmitters are relegated to the brain and spinal nerves, the microbiome of our gut that represents our inner Wei Qi strongly influences our moods, thoughts, and brain chemistry. The great majority of serotonin is found in the Wei Qi of the gut lining, which regulates the peristaltic waves of descending Stomach Qi, and variations can impact assimilation and absorption of the gastrointestinal (GI) tract. Constant bidirectional communication goes on between the gut and the brain. Not only does the vagus nerve (which runs along the Windows of Heaven points on the neck) communicate from the brain to the gut (as well as other organs), and back again, the gut is lined with over a hundred million nerve cells. That's because gut bacteria are busy producing neurotransmitters like serotonin, dopamine, norepinephrine, GABA, and acetylcholine. The specific blending of our gut bacteria determines aspects of our personality and sociability. When the body-mind experiences stress and resistance, so do the critters inhabiting our gut's inner landscape, producing bacteria that generate chemicals which cause immune-modulating and inflammatory mediators as well as mood disrupters responsible for symptoms of depression and anxiety. We can view this through the lens of the Small Intestine, whose job is to transmit the consciousness of the Heart into the gut. And part of the process of separating the pure from the impure is to illuminate all that is not in resonance with Heaven's mandate. In the darkness, light is cast on the shadows so they may release their hold on us. If we mask them, we may never walk the true path to our destiny, which is to find Heaven within, in all of its multifaceted expressions.

Our confusion begins when we use the limited and dualistic brain alone, the source of segmentation via Kidney Yin and Yang, to do the sorting according to our own separate will, which can never by itself bring us into alignment with our destiny. The tranquility of Heaven (also known as Reality) is always on offer, which only the Heart can receive. The Heart receives impressions and transmits them to the Lower Dan Tien, a process which allows for an ongoing alignment between the Heart and Kidneys and everything in between. Our feelings thus arise from within our Heart, gut, and heads.

We are meant to feel an array of feelings. The light of Shen vitalizes the Blood, allowing us to experience rises and falls of the Qi mechanism in response to the ever-changing weather of life. In states of elation, the Qi becomes loose. Obsessive thought knots the Qi. When there is anger, the Qi rises. Sadness causes the Qi to disappear, and fear makes the Qi descend. Ascendant Qi tends to increase excitatory neurotransmitters, and descending, fearful states will inhibit them. Frightful states cause the Qi to drastically descend, resulting in compensatory rises, disrupting communication between the Ministerial and Sovereign Fire. In our more sophisticated modern psyches, we experience emotional complexes such as shame, which causes the Qi to contract and disappear, and guilt, which takes the uprising strength of anger and contracts it inward, distorting other elemental movements with it. Yu 鬱, silt, describes a state of mental depression where a heavily laden head and Heart drag the legs along behind, hindering the free circulation of Qi, and blocking the light of Shen. Imagine what this will do to the neurotransmitters.

If our view of ourselves and life becomes imbalanced, thoughts, moods, and emotional states, along with their accompanying neurotransmitters, follow suit and become disordered. In these chaotic states, we are invited to be still, integrate, and thereby experience a new state of order, previously unknown, where we can occupy a new vibratory field with all of its offerings. Antidepressants and anxiolytics seek to manipulate the end result of the neurotransmitter's messages by hyper-stimulating deficient messages and calming hyperactivity, without causing a fundamental change in the individual's consciousness that would regulate them from the source and allow a new reality to emerge. According to our equation above, manipulating neurotransmitters is roughly at the Blood level, which is meant to follow the Qi. All true healing begins and ends in the Heart-Mind, which the Qi follows, and must allow Shen to enliven the Blood. We were meant to experience an array of thoughts and emotions, but not to become lost in them. The Spirit homes to a quiet Heart that can observe all mental and emotional states, while it follows the quiet urgings of the truth within.

Depression

Depression isn't a thing in itself, nor is it caused by a chemical imbalance. It is a state of deprivation caused by the maligned energies we have described, resulting in feelings other than those experienced by an unclouded Heart: quiet unconditional joy, love, and peace. The majority of us do not experience this state. Part of the reason for this is societal; humanity itself seems to be suffering from mental illness and the prognosis isn't good. Medication is unlikely to be the answer.

The first *Diagnostic and Statistical Manual of Mental Disorders* (DSM), printed as a 32-page spiral bound pamphlet in 1952, listed just over a hundred psychiatric disorders. Today's *DSM-5-TR* is 947 pages long and classifies three times as many mental illnesses, each with its own diagnostic code.

A high percentage of our population is being treated for depression, and prescriptions for antidepressants, antipsychotics, and anxiolytics are on the rise. This state of crisis has caused unprecedented rises in mental health admissions, with very little recovery. Whether or not people are actually more depressed now than ever before, prescriptions for antidepressants have increased. In July 2022, *The Pharmaceutical Journal* reported that antidepressant prescribing has increased 35 percent in six years (Royal Pharmaceutical Society, 2022). While the average age of those diagnosed with depression is 48 years of age, in 2021, 17 percent of college students were found to be taking antidepressants. In 2020, one-third of those prescribed antidepressants had no history of depression before receiving their prescription. Every year, doctors write hundreds of millions of prescriptions for antidepressants and benzodiazepines, and in one recent trial, only about half of the patients got any better, while many just experienced the side effects without any benefits. These are the symptoms of a collective mindset that is desolate, desperate, and looking for relief from the pain of being emotionally alive. Instead, they are lulled into a system that profits greatly by promising happiness but delivering varying states of emotional numbness. If we step out of compliance with this system of avoidance and instead feel our pain, we may actually become empowered to change the system that perpetuates it.

The most common symptoms of depression are feeling empty, sad, and hopeless. Depression can cause glucocorticoid resistance, increase levels of pro-inflammatory cytokines, and weaken the immune system. Common accompanying patterns include deficiencies in Kidney Qi, Spleen Qi, and Lung Qi, as well as Liver Qi stagnation and Heart Qi and Blood deficiency. Yu opposes the springing up of Wood in the Liver, and hinders the transformation function of Spleen Yang. When the Earth spirit, Yi, is injured, the mind can no longer give shape to images, and one cannot find purpose in anything and becomes disturbed almost to the point of complete disorder. The resulting havoc in the system will tempt us to do almost anything for relief.

Because the Liver wants to store things, it can store insults, resentments, hurt, and anger, stagnating the Qi and Blood. This is one of the reasons the Liver has the most points to rectify Qi, so we can release past insults. If we don't mend our relationship with past insults, we will keep producing situations to try to mend our past. Not only will this produce depressive states, it will not allow the Liver to generate vital new plans. Instead of numbing to them, we can use the Liver channel to forgive, allow rectification, and move on.

The Sinew channels are the first line of defense against outer aggressions, and often retain traumatic memories in the microfibers of the musculature, constituting a major part of our underlying belief patterns that result in subconscious posturing. This blocks the free flow of Qi and Blood, resulting in pain from stagnant holding patterns. Since antidepressants force the Qi to rise to the surface, some chronic pain conditions respond to antidepressants, although the source isn't resolved.

When the Qi mechanism is stifled through unfulfilled desires, conscious suppression, or unconscious repression, the Shen, Hun, and Po become disconnected, resulting in fatigue, sullenness, anxiety, restlessness, and absent mindedness. The resulting tension will need to be disinhibited through points such as Lv 3, Lv 14, GB 13, GB 34, GB 37, SJ 3, and Pc 6. When the depressed Qi results in Heat, it can injure the Kidney Yin or cause Heart Fire, for which Ht 7, Ht 8, or Ki 3 may help. When the Liver overacts on the Spleen, this can lead to Dampness and Phlegm, which may bind the chest or obstruct the orifices. Open the chest with GB 22, Sp 21, Lu 1, Lv 14, or Pc 6. Use Gua Sha around the diaphragm and intercostal areas. Formulas include Yue Ju Wan, Chai Hu Shu Gan Tang, and Si Ni San when extremities are cold, Xiao You San for deficient presentations, and Jia Wei Xiao Yao San if Heat is present. When

Heart Qi stagnates, palpitations and chest oppression worsen. Add Ren 15 or Ren 17, upper Kidney points, Ht 5 or Ht 7, and use Mu Xiang Liu Qi Yin. Depression due to Lung Qi stagnation will often include chest oppression, sighing, sadness, and shortness of breath, and may include anxiety. Lu 7, St 40, Ren 16, and Pc 6 can help resolve this, along with Ban Xia Huo Po Tang. A certain type of depression characterized by fatigue, shortness of breath, drowsiness, and a general lack of interest in life can be due to Spleen Qi deficiency. If the moods are prolapsed, St 36 and Du 20 along with Bu Zhong Yi Qi Tang can ascend the Qi to uplift the emotions.

Dietary modifications can remove Dampening foods from the diet, especially junk foods, fried foods, sugar, flour, refined carbohydrates, and highly processed foods laden with preservatives, which can all have a mood-dulling effect on the body-mind. Sometimes the easiest remedies are right in front of us. Fruits and vegetables may be nature's best antidepressant. Exposure to sunlight, and outdoor exercise to move and disinhibit the Qi mechanism, also help to raise neurotransmitter levels.

Another healing modality that helps with mild depression and anxiety is meditation. Most traditional healing methods encourage us to face our pain in order to overcome psychological suffering rather than masking it. A study reported in *Science Advances* in 2017 looked at the cognitive changes in meditators (Valk *et al.*, 2017). Breathing meditations with interoceptive body awareness provided moderate brain changes in the meditators. Perspective meditations, where one observed their thoughts, provided intermediate effects. The greatest mental and emotional changes diagnosed with magnetic resonance imaging (MRI) were experienced in those practicing loving kindness meditations, taking in the suffering of self and others. We are meant to take ourselves in rather than reject the parts of us we don't love. This is a big undertaking, especially when we see how vast we really are. When we can allow Shen to occupy the throne of the Heart, we can begin to identify with the peaceful witnessing quality of awareness, and let the Qi of depression, sadness, and hurt flow through us, rather than defining us.

The character for Gallbladder 胆囊 shows a person in a precarious position bent over a cliff, hesitant, yet needing to make the correct decision—with the courage, bravery, and strength that can only emerge with the necessary force that comes from an unshakably tranquil center. Only when the Gallbladder acts decisively can the 11 other officials respond accordingly. When a decision is made, the Gallbladder's uprising power bursts forth to open new possibilities, increases our levels of consciousness and clarity, and provides the courage to step into the pressure of whatever feels threatening, without allowing the fear of the unknown to hold us back. Sometimes it takes the bitterness of bile to digest fatty, lethargic states. The strength of the Gallbladder is able to overcome the contraction of fear so perverse qi cannot attack.

This is how distress can be converted into a challenge, helping us evolve. Stress responses are fabricated emotional constructions of the world, based on conditioning. The brain then predicts responses that will trigger this same emotional response (shame, fear, anxiety, etc.). We can view "stress" as negative and avoid it at all costs, or we can accept its presence as the physiological experience of transformation—as we approach a new challenge, we rise above previously held limitations and are made anew. The body may still feel anxious, but this is often necessary in accepting the freedom of new movement. The immune system is bolstered through short-term stressors. It's only when they're ongoing, without a push forward into new behavior, that the stress becomes chronic, where it increases cortisol and weakens the immune system. When we retreat in self-deprecation instead, stress hormones still increase, but they have no outlet.

While it might fly in the face of modern therapeutic techniques, I have walked with quite a few patients into and through their deepest psychic suffering, which previously had brought them to the point of suicidal despair. The only thing they had ever been offered before was talk therapy and mind-altering pharmaceuticals, which actually kept them back from the cliff, the verge of transformation. Only when you have befriended your own inner hauntings, however, can you walk with another through theirs. Then you can help them look into their darkest fears while tonifying the Kidneys; help them face their anger as you harmonize the Liver; support them as they release their grief while tonifying the Lungs; and overcome their obsessive worry through strengthening the Spleen. As they are able to scour the orifices of the heart, their Pericardium opens, and you may witness the reclamation of their inherent joy. Question your patients about their desire to get well, while checking the appearance of their Shen as they answer. If they say they are hopeful but their eyes become dull and their spirit leaves, perhaps there is a secondary gain in remaining unwell. Sometimes illness allows them to be seen and cared for in a way that wellness would not. Our remedies may not be able to reach them until they recognize these complicating obstructions.

We cannot heal the body if we leave the mind out, and we cannot heal the mind if we leave the body out. The first step is to fast from external distractions and overstimulation so we may bear witness to our own mental patterns. Ki 9 Guest House can help us step outside our patterns to bear witness to who we are. As we sit with ourselves and observe from within, we occupy the source, the original Chong Mai, where we can turn to the dynamics of the Ren Mai and ask what gives us a sense of comfort, bonding, and nourishment. Then we can look at the things we're sitting with that we shouldn't, that may accumulate and obstruct the Du Mai and overflow into the Dai Mai.

We all are prone to states of possession at times when subconscious energies take over our consciousness. We curse ourselves with negative self-talk, which may have come from past or ancestral voices. Long-term emotions and the thoughts that accompany them can become habitual, until our very identity depends on them, and changing ourself can be quite threatening. The hurtful effects may seem overwhelming, but we can invite the same ancestors to assist us in our transformation with SI 11. If the patient is open to change, focus on the original blueprint contained in the Chong Mai with Sp 4, encounter past conflicts held in the Yin Wei Mai with Pc 6, and the celestial chimney at Ren 22 to help them question their narratives. Lv 14 can activate past memories, and Sp 16 can address past regrets that have gone latent.

As individuals encounter the misunderstandings of the past, an inner unraveling may occur. Latent issues come out of their hiding place (like the Divergents, Dai Mai or Qiao Mai), and spread throughout the system. When the unconscious becomes conscious, these lurking Gui-like hauntings must be encountered, and the patient may initially feel worse about themselves rather than better. This is temporary; as they continue to circulate through the Blood, they can meet the light of Shen in the middle Dan Tien; the upper Dan Tien shifts its viewpoint, and the Po are allowed to exit. Treatment principles include helping to anchor them in their source as you release areas of holding like the hips, shoulders, and diaphragm. Internal questions that can guide them during treatments can include questions such as: What hurts your Heart most? What are your greatest regrets? Do you carry any secrets you've revealed to no one? When do you remember life as good? Are you living according to who you authentically are, or who you think you should be according to others? Are you dependent on anyone or anything for your emotional needs? If the psychic sclerosis isn't too severe, their Heart may open, and as Qi flow increases through the chest, Pc 8 may warm up.

While the scientific approach seeks to divide and separate in order to identify the problem and form the correct diagnoses, the entire method is based on the premise of entropy. The most radical healing, though, is based on integration. If we remain present to our discomfort without trying to manipulate it, the tension in the system can actually catalyze transformation to a higher level of organization. If our intention is primarily to relieve the discomfort of the tension, we may be depriving the individual of the transformative fuel necessary for the Shen to reach the constitutional level and transmute it.

Antidepressants

Antidepressants seek to provide an artificial means to enhance one's mood. We live in a very Yang society and interact with it in ways that often deplete the Yang Qi, exhausting the Liver and Heart's ability to harmonize with the external and internal worlds. We are often Yin and Blood deficient. The Liver may become overwhelmed, inhibiting the Qi mechanism, overacting on the Spleen, and further depleting our underlying reserves. Antidepressants intend to modulate the effects of neurotransmitters, resulting in relatively constant stimulation that enhances the Yang actions of the neurotransmitters at the synaptic junction. Many individuals diagnosed with depression are under the impression that they have a "chemical imbalance" that causes them to feel the way they do, which needs to be corrected with antidepressants. This is a very simplistic explanation for a complex situation that allows physicians to quickly write a prescription, without dealing with the underlying cause of the imbalance and sending patients on their way. Antidepressants may help patients feel better temporarily, and can be supportive during major life crises. Yet medical research abounds with examples of the limited effectiveness of antidepressants, which nonetheless does not seem to curtail their use.

Major classes of antidepressants include selective serotonin reuptake inhibitors (SSRIs), selective norepinephrine reuptake inhibitors (SNRIs), tricyclic antidepressants (TCAs), monoamine oxidase inhibitors (MAOIs), and atypical antidepressants that don't fit neatly into the other categories.

SSRIs

- Citalopram (Celexa)
- Escitalopram (Lexapro, Cipralex)
- Fluoxetine (Prozac, Oxactin)
- Fluvoxamine (Faverin)
- Paroxetine (Paxil, Pexeva)
- Sertraline (Zoloft, Lustral)
- Vortioxetine (Brintellix)
- Dapoxetine (Priligy)

SSRIs increase the duration of time that serotonin occupies the receptor site. While they provide the feeling of lifting the Yang Qi, they do not tonify. Instead, they simulate a lifting effect by activating Kidney Yang to raise Liver Yang, causing serotonin to remain longer at the synaptic cleft to stimulate the postsynaptic cellular membrane rather than moving it through. This process of overusing the Yang Qi has the effect of Dampening the natural movement of Qi, and can deplete the Blood. Side effects include impotence, erectile dysfunction, or lack of sexual desire, and rebellious Qi signs such as nausea, vomiting, insomnia, dizziness, headaches, hypertension, tachycardia, and photosensitivity. This constant barrage of Qi can also stimulate the Wei Qi sufficient to result in nervous system overactivity, while Dampening the Ming Men Fire.

Inhibiting reuptake of serotonin can cause accumulation and stagnation of fluids in both the Kidneys and Sea of Marrow. Ascending the Qi may be more problematic in those with pre-existing ascendant Liver Yang, as well as those with underlying Blood, Kidney, or Yuan Qi deficiencies. Side effects from SSRI withdrawal correlate with collapse of Yang, along with Qi stagnation, Spleen Qi deficiency, Liver Blood deficiency, Dampness, Blood stasis, and Shen disturbance. Again, we were meant to feel an array of feelings, not just one or two. Patients on antidepressants often feel unable to grieve losses fully because the Qi is unable to descend along with the circumstances. When working with someone on SSRIs we may need to anchor the Yang Qi, and subdue ascending Liver Yang. Formulas like Chai Hu Jia Long Gu Mu Li Tang are used precisely for this purpose. We may also need to drain Dampness and tonify the Blood. If we are helping someone wean off of them, we may need to take over lifting the Qi with points such as St 36, Ht 7, and Du 20, along with formulas like Bu Zhong Yi Qi Tang, if the underlying pattern includes Spleen Qi and Yang deficiency with collapse of Qi. Of course, pay attention to the actual presenting pattern and prescribe the appropriate tonifying and/or moving formula.

SNRIs

- Duloxetine (Cymbalta, Irenka, Drizalma Sprinkle)
- Desvenlafaxine (Pristiq, Khedezla)
- Venlafaxine (Effexor, Effexor XR)
- Milnacipran (Savella)
- Levomilnacipran (Fetzima)

In addition to increasing serotonin, SNRIs enhance the length of time norepinephrine stimulates the receptor sites. SNRIs have the effect of lifting the Qi due to the serotonin-enhancing effects; side effects are like SSRIs, but norepinephrine more strongly ascends Yang. SNRIs are more stimulating than SSRIs, and initial side effects are due to serotonin stimulation, while subsequent side effects include dry mouth and night sweats. Kidney Yang may lose its anchoring and float upwards, overacting on the surface and upper part of the body. Kidney Yin may become deficient, fluids may stagnate, ascendant Liver Yang and Wind may result, and the Hun and Shen may be disturbed, depleting Liver and Heart Yin, and eventually Kidney Yang. Therefore, our treatments might include tonifying Kidney Yin, anchoring Kidney Yang, and clearing Liver Heat, as well as disinhibiting the Qi mechanism which may have caused the depression in the first place.

TCAs

- Amitriptyline (Elavil, Vanatrip)
- Doxepin (Silenor, Sinequan)
- Clomipramine (Anafranil)
- Nortriptyline (Pamelor)
- Imipramine (Tofranil)
- Desipramine (Norpramin)
- Protriptyline (Vivacity)
- Amoxapine (Asendin)
- Trimipramine (Surmontil)

Tricyclic antidepressants block the reuptake of monoamine neurotransmitters dopamine, norepinephrine, and serotonin, causing elevated synaptic levels of these feel-good neurotransmitters. Sometimes more effective than the previous classes, they can flood the synapses and are often used to treat major depression episodes along with panic attacks, obsessive compulsive disorders, and suicidal thoughts. Commensurate with their therapeutic effect of raising Liver Yang, they also exhibit a greater array of side effects, including nausea, flu-like symptoms, and mania, but their Dampening effect can also produce symptoms like sedation, lethargy, orthostatic hypotension, hypomania, weight gain, and impotence. In addition, anticholinergic effects like dry mouth, urinary retention, and decreased bowel motility result. The Yang stimulation depletes Stomach Yin and impairs fluid metabolism. This can dampen Yang Ming, exhaust Spleen Yang, and lead to Dampness, but can also result in Yang Ming Heat.

MOAIs

- Phenelzine (Nardil)
- Tranylcypromine (Parnate)
- Selegiline (Eldepryl, Emsam, Zelapar)
- Isocarboxazid (Marplan)

Monoamine oxidase inhibitors block the metabolism of serotonin, norepinephrine, and dopamine, increasing their synaptic concentration. Used in more resistant depression, panic, and social disorders, they strongly stimulate the central nervous system, producing side effects such as orthostatic hypotension, hepatotoxicity, agitation, hyperreflexia, blood pressure alterations, and, at high doses, hallucinations and convulsions. They also suppress rapid eye movement (REM) sleep. Because MOAIs inhibit certain enzymes, dietary modifications are required, such as eliminating tyramine-rich foods like aged cheese, animal liver, salami, alcohol, and soy sauce, to avoid developing a hypertensive crisis. They strongly ascend Yang, potentially to the point of unrooting the Hun. Again, our treatment principles may need to anchor the Yang, restore the up-down dynamic, harmonize the Liver, and root the Hun.

Atypical antidepressants

- Bupropion (Wellbutrin, Zyban)
- Mirtazapine (Remeron)
- Vilazodone (Viibryd)
- Vortioxetine (Trintellix, Brintellix)
- Trazodone (Desyrel)
- Nefazodone (Serzone)

Atypical antidepressants are simply those that act in ways that don't fall into the above four categories. Some inhibit the reuptake of dopamine, others boost serotonin levels by other means. Wellbutrin, for example, blocks the reuptake of norepinephrine and dopamine, while leaving serotonin intact. It also impacts nicotine receptors and thus can help reduce cravings. While its Yang-invigorating effects may help course the Qi, the ascending quality gives rise to side effects like hypertension, anxiety, headache, and dizziness, induced by resultant Wind and Heat. Like Chai Hu, this Yang effect may also produce Dryness, which can lead to constipation. Constant stimulation of the neurotransmitters doesn't harmonize the Qi, per se, but can overstimulate the Yang, potentially resulting in Yin and Blood deficiency, especially at higher doses. The body may then compensate for the Yin vacuity by holding on to Dampness. Serzone exhibits similar side effects, as well as weight loss, hypotension, and erectile dysfunction. Liver damage may also result, hence Serzone was withdrawn from other countries although is still prescribed in the United States. Deseryl causes more drowsiness due to its Dampening qualities and is often prescribed for insomnia. Remeron, which affects Stomach Qi, has more anxiolytic qualities due to its more Dampening effects, resulting in increase in appetite, weight gain, and can lower white blood cell counts. Its ability to disrupt the Qi mechanism can also cause glaucoma, heart rhythm abnormalities, and seizures. Atypical antidepressants are often prescribed after the other classes have not been effective at resolving the issues. This class might be more effective for smoking cessation, bulimia, or seasonal affective disorder.

Most antidepressants take two to four weeks to exhibit their full effects, during which time some younger patients under age 25, with more Yang, tend to experience increase in suicidal thoughts and behaviors. This tells us that the increased Yang stimulation can exacerbate the underlying emotional reactivity. Over time, the individual tends to acclimate to these symptoms, but emotional highs and lows are muted. Patients on antidepressants tend to have a glazed look in their eyes instead of the healthy illumination of Shen. Many report they don't feel their emotions as much, as the vulnerability of the Pericardium is reduced in its capacity to connect to the feeling states of the Heart, and it is more difficult to cry. GB 41 may be able to help them release their tears as the emotions which are held latent in the Dai Mai are liberated.

Keep in mind that our treatments won't be able to overcome the effects of the antidepressants while they are taking them, but we should always tonify what's weak, and resolve any excess. When treating patients taking Yang-invigorating drugs, their fluids and blood should be monitored and supplemented to moderate the side effects of the medication. Additionally, it may be useful to make sure the Yang Qi remains anchored and rooted. Monitoring blood pressure and other possible cardiac effects would be an important part of working with these patients.

Care must be taken when helping patients wean off of antidepressants as they can experience erratic movements of Qi, and flooding of emotions, but we can calm the Shen, restore the Heart-Kidney axis, harmonize the Qi, and address the underlying pattern of imbalance.

Now that we've covered the dynamics of pharmaceutical antidepressant medications, let's take a look at some natural substances that exert similar effects. St. John's Wort contains the active ingredient hypericin, which is charged with its ability to treat mild to moderate depression. Once the chemical compound responsible for its therapeutic effects has been isolated in a plant, it can be studied, concentrated, and used to induce specific physiological effects. Hypericin has been found to lift moods by increasing the levels of serotonin, norepinephrine, dopamine, GABA, and L-glutamine. Like many other adaptogens, it also contains immune-boosting properties that render it effective against viruses, bacteria, and fungal infections. St. John's Wort can produce side effects like GI upset, dry mouth, constipation, dizziness, and restlessness; and because of its immune-enhancing effects, it has been found to interfere with immunosuppressive drugs that prevent organ transplant rejection. Thus, we can infer that it stimulates and lifts the Yang Qi, making patients more resilient to their environment.

Further, Omega-3 EPA/DHA has been found to help serotonin molecules fit into the receptor sites on brain cell membranes. While it doesn't raise neurotransmitter levels, this Jing tonic helps to stabilize moods in part through its Yin-nourishing, Yang-anchoring effect.

5-hydroxytryptophan (5-HTP) is a metabolite of the amino acid tryptophan, a precursor to serotonin. Available as a supplement, 5-HTP can help restore serotonin levels, especially after being on antidepressants.

Weaning off antidepressants
Helping someone reduce or eliminate antidepressants may involve encountering and supporting people through potentially challenging psycho-emotional issues—not every practitioner's forte. Make sure you are comfortable addressing these concerns before you become part of their support team. Certain antidepressants like Effexor (cleverly nicknamed "side effexor") can cause rather extreme Shen-disturbing side effects when someone is weaning off them.

After receiving treatments for the second trajectory of the Chong Mai to address a bound Heart and Pericardium from childhood trauma,

Justin felt ready to go off his Effexor, a prescription he had been on for three years at 75 mg/day for depression and anxiety. He had tried to go off his medication before, and said he felt extremely agitated and crazy, and while not overtly suicidal, he could recognize and understand those tendencies now. This time, with his doctor's concurrence, we slowly weaned him off his prescription with Chinese medical support.

For his dosing schedule he reduced every other day's dosage by one half at certain increments. For example, on the first day, he took half a pill at 37.5 mg, followed the next day by his usual full tablet at 75 mg. Every other day he alternated, taking a full dose one day followed the next day with half a pill. He stayed at this dosage, averaging 50 mg/day for two weeks, during which time he experienced no side effects. He then cut back to 37.5 mg each day. After two weeks, he reduced his dosage every other day to 18.75 mg, taking half a pill one day, a quarter the next. Then he took a quarter pill every day, followed by a quarter pill every other day. (If the patient experiences any uncomfortable side effects, go back to the previous dose until they stabilize.)

The entire process took three months, during which time treatment principles included calming the Shen, harmonizing and lifting the Qi, and rooting the Hun, using points like Ht 7, Lv 8, Lv 14, Pc 6, Du 20, Yintang, and ear Shenmen. He also supplemented with 2000 mg fish oil, 50 mg 5-HTP sublingual, 20 mg lithium orotate to stabilize moods, and 900 mg St. John's Wort to increase serotonin levels. Eventually he came off St. John's Wort, during which time he received Chai Hu Jia Long Gu Mu Li Tang. Later he came off the herbs as well but continued to supplement with the fish oil and 5-HTP.

Amphetamines
Mixed amphetamine salts

- Adderall
- Mydayis
- Adzenys
- Vyvanse

Attention deficits often manifest with loose and scattered Qi, lacking consolidation. This may be caused by weakness in the Kidneys' ability to consolidate, or impairment of the Spleen's function of storing reflection and linking thoughts and ideas. The Spleen may be unable to perform its special function of remonstrating with the Emperor. The resulting weakness in the unroofed Heart causes the Shen to destabilize.

Any Heat in the system further agitates the Mind. Obsessive thoughts consume the Central Qi, making the Hun fly away without direction, and the Po stir about thoughtlessly. The Zhi and Yi lose the harmonization through which the mental world is constructed. Shen's inability to control the Hun is revealed by diminished activity in the prefrontal cortex in attention deficit disorder (ADD). Treatment involves clearing Heat, tonifying the Kidneys, Spleen, and Heart as needed, rooting the Hun, and encouraging the individual to remain attentive to their inner state, noticing their appetites for overstimulation and resisting the tendency to flit about from one interest to another.

While not considered antidepressants, stimulants like Adderall, containing mixed amphetamine salts, are prescribed to help those with attention deficit disorders to focus and concentrate; yet they also increase energy levels and moods, sometimes quite dramatically. Since their primary mode of action increases synaptic concentrations of serotonin, norepinephrine, and dopamine levels, they are sometimes prescribed off label for depression. Since the Covid-19 pandemic, prescriptions for Adderall have increased to the point that it became short in supply. While the evidence is mixed as to whether the recipients actually suffer from clinical depression, apathy, or boredom, a little pick-me-up can help one get a whole lot done. The mechanism is similar to SNRIs, only much stronger. They overly stimulate Kidney Yang to arouse Liver Yang, which can then disturb the Heart. While this burst of Yang energy can certainly rev up one's mood, such stimulants are very habit forming and carry a high risk of dependence. This is especially true for people who have histories of addictive tendencies, and those with attention deficit hyperactivity disorder (ADHD) have a greater risk of suicidal thoughts and behaviors while taking these medications.

Amphetamine salts obviously do not treat the source; while the stimulating effect can temporarily override the loose Qi mechanism, and Yang might pierce through some Phlegm obstruction, it does not correct it. The resulting Heat can produce headaches, insomnia, anxiety, psychotic episodes, and worsening depression. Amphetamines strongly invigorate and drain Kidney Yang and ascend Liver Yang, resulting in Liver or Heart Fire, fluid depletion, dryness, Kidney Yin and Yang deficiency, and Heat and Wind symptoms. Patients who are Yin deficient or those with patterns of Heat will assuredly suffer more agitating side effects from taking amphetamines than those with Phlegm obstruction or Yang deficiency.

Anxiety

We are an anxious society as we have to adapt to a hectic world we were not meant to inhabit without a strong inner anchor. Our thoughts tend to run wild as we experience increased levels of stress as the result of modern life. We work too many hours, and experience economic stress, relationship stress, stress of being alone, technology-induced anxiety, eco anxiety, and lack of the harmonizing effects of being in nature. Being self-medicating humans, we often drink alcohol and use tetrahydrocannabinol (THC) to calm us down.

Anxiety disorders, phobias, and panic attacks are mediated by hyperactivity of the sympathetic nervous system. The primary symptom of anxiety is a persistent and prevalent state of worry that persists for over six months. Other symptoms include muscular tension, fatigue, insomnia, irritability, and digestive disturbances. Panic attacks include more chest symptoms like palpitations, shortness of breath, chest pain, and choking sensation, with dizziness, trembling, fear of losing control, going crazy, or dying. Anxiety and palpitations can include patterns like Heart Blood, Yin, or Qi deficiency, along with other deficiencies and resulting excess. Treatment principles include nourishing the Heart, calming the mind, clearing Heat, resolving Phlegm, or invigorating Blood as the particular pattern indicates. Acupoints might include Ht 5, Ht 7, Ren 14, Ren 15, UB 15, UB 44, GB 13, UB 17, and Ki 22–27, among others, depending on the particular pattern. Common herbal formulas might include Gui Pi Tang, Tian Wan Bu Xin Dong, An Shen Ding Zhi Wan, Gui Shen Tang, or Wen Dan Tang. Anxiety and depression often go together, and sometimes when anxiety symptoms subside, there is an underlying deficient and depressed state behind it.

Anxiolytics

Anxiolytics all work in different ways, but these depressant medications all lower overall brain activity. More females take anti-anxiety medication, and the percentages increase to over 10 percent of the population in the post-menopausal years.

Benzodiazepines

- Alprazolam (Xanax)
- Chlordiazepoxide (Librium)
- Clonazepam (Klonopin)
- Clorazepate (Tranxene)
- Diazepam (Valium)
- Halazepam (Paxipam)
- Lorazepam (Ativan)
- Oxazepam (Serax)
- Prazepam (Centrax)
- Quazepam (Doral)

Benzodiazepines are central nervous system depressants that calm overstimulation by slowing messages to the brain, producing hypnotic states of calm and relaxation. Benzodiazepines bind GABA receptors, increasing chloride and driving it into the nerve cells. This reduces communication between brain cells to calm down the fight-flight response. This ends up producing a Dampening effect. Chloride is a halogen that retains heat, impeding the action of Kidney Yang and San Jiao, disrupting the Fire/Water balance, thus requiring a greater threshold to induce a response in the nervous system. This inhibits Wood and dampens Shao Yang; as a result, ascendant Yang is prevented from stirring the Heart, thus sedating the Heart Qi, Blood, and Shen. Benzodiazepines like Xanax actually shut off the amygdala, depressing Liver Qi functioning so we don't have to deal with pain. Side effects are due to the Qi's Stagnating and Dampening qualities, including loss of coordination, slowed breathing, blurred vision, stuffy nose, stomach and bowel changes, swelling of hands and feet, chest pain, lowered libido, reduced concentration and memory loss, irritability, fatigue, dependence, and severe withdrawal symptoms. Long-term use can cause Phlegm to obstruct the orifices of the Heart. There are three types of benzodiazepines: short, intermediate, and long acting. Short-acting drugs tend to be more addictive and cause more severe symptoms as one comes down from the drug. These types of medicines should be used symptomatically for short periods of time, to avoid dependence and strong effects of withdrawal.

Barbiturates

- Amobarbital (Amytal)
- Butabarbital (Butisol)
- Pentobarbital (Nembutal)
- Secobarbital (Seconal)
- Phenobarbital (Donnatal)
- Butalbital/acetaminophen/caffeine (Esgic, Fioricet)
- Butalbital/aspirin/caffeine (Fiorinal, Ascomp, Fortabs)

Barbiturates are sedative-hypnotic drugs that, like benzodiazepines, attempt to reduce anxiety by binding to GABA receptors to open the chloride channel in the GABA neurotransmitter. This has a strong effect of reducing nerve impulses, resulting in more sedating effects, drowsiness, and hypnosis. Side effects include dyspnea, confusion, fainting, bradycardia, dizziness, vertigo, hypothermia, and muscle weakness. They are very habit forming, and can result in death from overdose. Their effects are quite cooling and Dampening, and while their intended effect is to calm the Shen down, they often end up smothering it. Some are laced with pain relievers and caffeine to attempt to counter the sedating effects.

Anxiolytics relieve the sensation of anxiety, by "taking it away," but users report they take it *all* away. While the anxious, fearful feelings may subside, so do feelings of joy and connection. The person is often left feeling isolated and alone, with only their drug for comfort. Their expressions may be flat and they often exhibit a dullness of the eyes. Chinese medicine might aim at clearing Heart Heat, descending Liver Yang, and calming the Shen. We can support patients by resolving Phlegm, opening the orifices, harmonizing the Qi, and leading the Fire down. Herbal formulas like Chai Hu Jia Long Gu Mu Li Tang might be a therapeutic way to help patients reduce or cut out their reliance on anxiolytics. I always encourage meditation and other non-medicinal means like Qi Gong and body wisdom to find distance from the thoughts and emotions that get caught in the orifices of the Heart.

Insomnia

As you can see, many of the above drugs may alleviate insomnia, which is described as one of the symptoms of a Shen disturbance. Others, which lift the Qi, can contribute to or give rise to insomnia. We all want to have enough energy and vitality; we also need to return to a state of inner peace where we may return to the dark to be restored. The worlds we occupy can be very challenging, requiring great amounts of Qi and Blood to keep up with the demands we have placed on ourselves. This can leave us weary and exhausted, and yet too wired to rest fully and restore ourselves. Insomnia tends to worsen with age because as our Yin and Blood stores become depleted, the warm Wei Qi, which moves inward at night, can produce a harassing effect. In fact, almost one-third of older adults are prescribed sleeping pills. Revisiting Qi Bo's response to Huang Di as to why the elderly don't sleep well:

> The strong have an exuberance of Qi and Blood, they have fatty flesh and muscles, their pathways of Qi are unimpeded, and their Ying and Wei are without irregularity. Thus they are energetic by day and sleep at night. As for the old, their Qi and Blood are diminished, their flesh and muscles are with-ered, their pathways of Qi are astringed, *the Qi of the five viscera are in conflict with one another,* Ying Qi is decrepit and scant, and the Wei Qi harasses the interior. Thus by day they are not energetic and by night they cannot sleep.

We all know that poor sleep hygiene practices include working late, watching TV, streaming internet content, being on screens, and so on, while proper sleep hygiene practices enhance Yin states to encourage melatonin produc-tion after the sun sets. These include low lighting, meditating, reading by candlelight, drinking chamomile tea, and listening to soothing music. But rarely do we hear about making sure the Qi of the five viscera are not in conflict with one another so the Wei Qi won't harass the interior. This means we don't let the sun go down on our anger. We don't carry worry, fear, or regret into sleep. If the day isn't over in our minds, we may spend our precious resources toiling, strategizing, and overthinking, when we should be letting go into the great Yin's embrace. Insomnia can be an invitation for inner psychic resolution.

Common excess patterns associated with insomnia include Liver Qi stagnation transforming into Liver Fire, disturbance of Phlegm Heat, Hyperactivity of Fire due to Yin deficiency, and Heat in the Diaphragm. Deficient conditions, which are more often seen in chronic insomnia, include Heart and Spleen vacuity, Heart and Gallbladder vacuity, Heart Yin/Blood or Liver Yin/Blood vacuity, and disharmony between the Heart and Kidneys.

Sleep aids

Antihistamines like diphenhydramine and doxylamine cause drowsiness and can facilitate sleep by their Cold, drying, and sedating qualities, but they also cause dizziness, grogginess, and memory impairment. They are not recommended for individuals over 65 because they can contribute to the development of senile dementia.

Barbiturates and benzodiazepines have Dampening qualities that are commonly used to facilitate sleep, although they do not produce deep, restorative sleep states. Because of their risks of drowsiness and increased propensity for falls, doctors began to prescribe "Z" drugs like zolpidem (Ambien, Edluar), zaleplon (Sonata), and eszopiclone (Lunesta). These sedative hypnotic pharmaceuticals induce side effects like amnesia, hallucinations, and parasomnia. Many patients sleep walk, drive, have sex, and go internet shopping at night on these drugs without any memory of having done so. Falls, fractures, and motor vehicle accidents are not uncommon side effects experienced by the unrooted Hun as they wander around carrying unconscious bodies with them, albeit "asleep."

Orexin receptor antagonists suvorexant (Belsomra), lemborexant (Dayvigo), and daridorexant (Quiviviq) are also sedative hypnotics but reportedly have fewer side effects than the Z drugs and are less habit forming, but they are also expensive. Side effects include decreased alertness and grogginess during the day, headaches, depression, sleep paralysis, and hallucinations.

While these drugs are Cold and have a Dampening effect, their Phlegm-like effects on consciousness obstruct the orifices of the Heart and unroot the Hun, which seem to wander around aimlessly, and do not allow for the necessary deep restorative sleep. Patterns like Liver Fire, diaphragm Heat, and Phlegm Fire harassing the Heart may tend to be worsened by the Phlegm-inducing effects of these pharmaceuticals. Our treatment principles will need to address the underlying pattern, which may include Kidney and Liver Yin deficiency and Liver and/or Heart Blood deficiency, while resolving Phlegm and Dampness and reinvigorating and rooting the Yang.

Bipolar disorder

Bipolar disorder is characterized by alternating periods of mania and depression. Chinese medicine refers to this disorder as Dian Kuang, caused by Phlegm misting the mind, obscuring the relationship between Shen, Hun, and Po. During times of elation, moods are elevated and expansive. Heat agitates the Hun, causing hyperactive, impulsive behavior, the Qi is loose, and the Shen scatters and is unable to keep the Hun in check.

After periods of uncontrolled elation, the spirits may then plunge into the depths, where the Po become disturbed, causing anxious, depressive, and hopeless moods, fatigue, loss of pleasure in life, and suicidal thoughts. Treatment principles are to calm the Shen (Chai Hu Jia Long Gu Mu Li Tang), and address underlying patterns of Phlegm misting the Mind (Ban Xia Huo Po Tang), Heart and Liver Fire (Long Dan Xie Gan Tang), disinhibit Liver Qi stagnation (Xiao Yao San, Xiao Chai Hu Tang), or Heart and Gallbladder deficiency (Ding Zhi Wan). St 40, Pc 6, GB 13, UB 44, UB 47, Ht 3, Ht 7, Du 20, Sp 6, St 45, and Ki 1 are appropriate acupoints from which to choose.

Treatment principles may also include helping patients to honor their process rather than strictly pathologizing it. Think of the Stomach's relationship to the intestinal flora and its ability to influence our mood states through the gut's neurotransmitters. One of the indications for the Jing Well point of leg Yang Ming St 45 is to address scenarios characterized by such expressions as *desiring to ascend to high places and sing, discard clothing and run around.* I am reminded of Lalla, the 14th-century mystic who uttered, "My teacher told me one thing: *Live in the soul.* When that was so, I began to go naked and dance." Severe mood fluctuations may not belong in orderly societal constructs, but it seems as if some souls long for extremes.

Antipsychotics

- Haloperidol (Haldol)
- Loxapine (Loxitane)
- Olanzapine (Zyprexa)
- Aripiprazole (Abilify)
- Risperidone (Risperdal)
- Quetiapine (Seroquel)
- Caripraszine (Vraylar)
- Lumateperone (Caplet)
- Lurasidone (Latuda)
- Asenapine (Saphris)
- Ziprasidone (Geodon)
- Fluoxetine with olanzapine (Symbol)
- Samidorphan with olanzapine (Lybalvi)
- Quetiapine fumarate (Seroquel)

Antipsychotics, also known as neuroleptics, are typically prescribed for schizophrenia, but are also scripted off label to manage severe bipolar disorder. They reduce the symptoms of delusions and hallucinations, anxiety, agitation, mania, confusion, and violent behavior, features that correlate with disturbed Shen and Hun. The patterns associated with these presentations are dominated by Heart and Liver Fire and Phlegm Heat. Antipsychotics can cause weakness, headaches, dizziness, dry mouth, and weight gain. Antipsychotic therapies that blanket the Shen often involve a cooling and Dampening mechanism which can disrupt fluid metabolism and obstruct the orifices, resulting in sedation, blurred vision, and impaired movement. We could help by calming the Shen and rooting the Hun while ameliorating some of the side effects by tonifying the Qi, transforming Dampness, and resolving Phlegm. Antipsychotics are often prescribed at end of life to prevent agitation and anxiety associated with the dying process. Unfortunately, though, these drugs tend to smother the Shen, which has a whole host of complications for the Yang spirits as they are passing through the death portal.

Mood stabilizers

- Carbamazepine (Carbatrol, Epitol, Equetro, Tegretol)
- Divalproex sodium (Depakote)
- Lamotrigine (Lamictal)
- Valproic acid (Depakene)
- Lithium carbonate (Lithobid)

Mood stabilizers are a class of drugs that act within the cell to treat manic episodes by modulating the activity of enzymes, ion channels, and arachidonic acid turnover, among others. While each has a slightly different mode of action, they all aim to decrease brain activity to reduce mood swings. Carbamazepine (Carbatrol, Epitol, Equetro, Tegretol), lamotrigine (Lamictal), and divalproex sodium (Depakote) are anticonvulsants that decrease nerve impulses. They can also stagnate the Blood, and weaken the Kidney and Liver. These mood stabilizers can steady the Shen and temporarily root the Hun, but can overly sedate, causing drowsiness, weakness, coordination difficulty, blurred or double vision, and weight gain. Here our treatment principles may include tonifying the Kidneys and Liver, calming the Shen, rooting the Hun, invigorating the Blood, resolving Dampness and Phlegm obstructing the orifices of the Heart, lifting clear Yang, and descending turbid Yin.

Lithium is a mineral salt found naturally in saline basins, bedrock, and clay beds. Minerals are settling and have anchoring properties. Lithium carbonate is a commonly prescribed mood stabilizer with a relatively narrow therapeutic window and hefty side effects from nausea, diarrhea, increased urination, and dry mouth to hypothyroid and renal toxicity. Patients with bipolar disorder often exhibit other pro-inflammatory cytokines, and lithium has been found to reduce neuroinflammation, which can contribute to depression. Lithium carbonate is a toxic drug which has to be closely monitored. It has a cooling and drying effect, which slows the firing of the nervous system, but can also damage Kidney Yang and the San Jiao mechanism. Lithium orotate is considered a dietary supplement, and is thus obtainable without a prescription. While low doses exert the same Shen stabilizing effects as lithium carbonate, the orotate form is proposed to cross the blood brain barrier more efficiently, has less renal toxicity, and actually promotes the regrowth of nerve cells in the hippocampus. Lithium seems to anchor the frantic comings and goings of an unrooted Hun, as it reduces excitatory neurotransmitters and increases GABA's inhibitory effects. It also subdues norepinephrine, and can have an antagonistic effect on thyroid hormone. Keep the Windows of Heaven open.

Barbara, a woman in her late thirties, was married a second time to a man, just like her first husband, who treated her poorly. This triggered her sense of insignificance, and she didn't feel capable of encountering the feelings of failure from another broken marriage. Sad, depressed, and anxious, she sought help from her doctor, who prescribed Elavil, a tricyclic antidepressant. She felt better within a couple of weeks, and stayed in the marriage three more years. As the abuse worsened, she of course felt worse and complained to her doctor about her worsening depression, now compounded by anxiety. Her dosage was increased, and she was also prescribed Xanax for her newly diagnosed panic disorder. As she became increasingly confused and disoriented, she finally sought help from a therapist, who supported her until she was able to leave the marriage. Eventually, with the added help of Chinese medicine, she was able to wean herself off her medication. She wasn't ever "clinically depressed"; the anguish she was experiencing was because she was being prompted to make a change that she resisted. She holds the antidepressant responsible for staying in the marriage to sustain the mounting physical and emotional injuries over the intervening years. But she learned a tremendous amount through her process, and claims she will never again resort to pharmaceutical means to remedy her life lessons.

Final thoughts

As you help resolve the symptoms associated with mood disorders, always look to the root. For while we can often make someone feel better, true healing sometimes happens when we no longer find the need to try to fix things in place. Only in states of acceptance do we become receptive to transformation. This, however, requires the courage to step out of past conditioning and surrender to the pure potential of the great unknown. We have to approach those tormented by grave psychological difficulties with great love and concern, and not take their difficulties lightly. But the root of that which plagues our psyches often stems from failure to love ourselves enough to bear witness to who we really are, where we are going, and who is in charge of our destiny.

While Chinese medicine is fully capable of treating psychological disorders, I encourage practitioners to work at this level only when they are confident in their own skills and have done their own "shadow work" so that they can walk with another who is encountering theirs. Whether someone has received a diagnosis of a psychological disorder described by the prevailing collective medical thought system or not, we all need help and support at times to find and live in the soul so our emotions don't overwhelm us.

This level of work can challenge whether or not our blueprint, ascribed by Heaven, is in alignment with the way we walk in the world. Some of the inner narratives we grapple with may originate from messages we've absorbed from ancestors, parents, friends, and other significant people in our lives who give us our beliefs about who we are. These beliefs give rise to the roles we inhabit, which may be at odds with our Chong Mai, but we don't know who we'd be without them. This is especially true during the cycles of seven and eight, when Jing makes itself available for realignment, when our sense of self is meant to destabilize. We often need to be shaken out of our slumber in order to get back on our true paths of awakening. Anything less isn't the Tao. We may be carrying unexamined hauntings from lessons we haven't yet learned or regrets we haven't forgiven. The seven Po, emissaries of the Queen Mother of the West, are often lurking just below the level of consciousness. Our work here is to support the patient as they face and examine the source of their suffering, rather than muting their discomfort, so they may consciously overcome worn-out ways of being. Suffering can be the gateway for the light to transform the darkness. If we don't resist what is by our attempts to manipulate life, the Mysterious Mother can reach in and offer her sometimes terrible, but always effective, cure. For the Mysterious Mother lives not on the mountain peak, but in the Spirit of the Valley, the doorway through which Heaven and Earth mingle, as she beckons us ever deeper into the Mysterious Pass, where the descent becomes the portal to one's ascent. While we may feel we've lost our way, we are never not home. While we may feel broken, if we allow ourselves to let go and break open, we might just make room for our souls to inhabit their rightful place in the realm of Heaven on Earth.

CHAPTER 5

Pain and Pain Relievers

Stay in the center,
even when there is pain.
Saying yes to our pain allows us to
say yes to the happiness underneath.

When I was first introduced to Chinese medicine, I was fascinated with the practice of Qi Gong. I read books, practiced on my own, and found the very few teachers who taught in my area. A martial arts academy in our local Chinatown held Tai Qi and Qi Gong classes, in which I immediately enrolled. We did not start out practicing the elegant movements I expected, but instead held challenging poses for inordinate amounts of time. During one class, we were instructed on how to do "neck stands" (headstands with our necks tucked forward), which I found quite difficult. After a grueling few minutes, my neck and upper back became quite uncomfortable, and I grimaced and grunted to show my discontent, hoping the instructor would come over and help me. He finally did come over, looked down at my twisted facial expression, and said "It's only pain" and walked away. I was stunned. *Only* pain?! I could barely even take in the bizarre suggestion that pain was merely an interpretation. I have since learned to appreciate his wisdom, and that pain can be observed without overly involving or identifying myself with it.

A couple years later, I was interning at a hospital in China, where I gingerly inserted needles with guide tubes so the patients wouldn't experience discomfort. Not only did they not experience discomfort, they didn't experience the Da Qi sensation they were used to. One patient looked at my attending physician, shook his head, and said *Méi yǒu*, or "No." She responded by removing me from his care and taking over his treatment. She then offered me one long needle and said when I was able to put it through my notebook, I could try needling again. And that's all I did for two or three days, until I was finally able to direct the Qi through the book without inner resistance, and it emerged through the hundreds of pages and poked out of the back cover. I had a new respect for the needle, and no longer feared causing pain. The next time I tried on a patient, the needle, as an extension of my Qi, shot directly into the point, and he felt the Da Qi without the skin's pain receptors being activated. Sometimes it takes a bit of discomfort to alleviate pain. That is not a popular idea in our society, and perhaps one of the reasons acupuncture isn't used as a first modality, although I hope and suspect that this will be happening for a greater majority. Healing is sometimes painful, representing a call to pay attention to something which we haven't acknowledged. We haven't learned how to be with our aches and pains, which has made for a very lucrative industry in covering up the manifestations of our discomfort.

While more safeguards have been applied to stop the rampant prescriptions for controlled substances to treat pain, the foundations of the system itself haven't changed. The "opioid crisis" continues, killing hundreds every day. We simply cannot afford, it seems, to put the brakes on an industry that generates such enormous profits. And the system can't be separated from its consumers: "The Man" has children. And these offspring, like the Sackler heirs, go about attempting to alleviate their discomfort rather than heeding the collective wake-up call.

The annual cost of treating pain conditions through the US health care industry has reached approximately 300 billion dollars. Epidemiological studies estimate that more than one quarter of our population, over 100 million Americans, are affected by chronic pain, and in addition to the medical cost, they spend about 30 billion dollars on complementary modalities to address their pain conditions that biomedicine hasn't been able to resolve. The United States is third on the list of painkiller consumption, with Germany leading the way, followed by Iceland; Canada is close behind the US. Oxycodone is the most heavily consumed controlled opioid, followed by morphine and methadone.

Because the perception of pain is so subjective, very few clinical findings can provide diagnostic certainty as to the source of pain, and how to alleviate it. Dolorology is the study of the origin, nature, and management of pain, and "pain management" has become its own board-certified medical specialty. While pain management physicians perform interventional procedures like nerve blocks and spinal cord stimulators, the bulk of their practice hours are spent doling out pharmaceuticals to manage chronic pain.

Pain is a helpful and necessary subjective experience based on signals the body experiences to help it maneuver away from noxious or harmful stimuli. Individual response to pain signals is a very complex process, and varies greatly based on the history and background of the particular pain condition, each person's unique emotional makeup, and the sensitivity of their nervous systems. Basically, pain is experienced when sensations at a certain locale are transmitted through the spinal cord to the brain where they are processed by the limbic system, thalamus, somatosensory cortex of the parietal lobe, and the prefrontal region. Pain is then experienced through the four processes of:

- transduction—mechanical, heat, or chemical stimuli activate afferent nociceptors in the tissues
- transmission—the pain signal travels from the periphery to the central nervous system via the spinal cord
- modulation—the pain signal is filtered by the brain, and transmitted to the somatosensory cortex where the pain is localized and emo-tionalized and instructions are sent back to the body part that signals how to react
- perception—the pain is perceived based on biological, psychological, and social factors.

Pain receptors are specific for the type of information they convey. Some report cold, some heat, and others let us know that there is a breach in the skin. Touch is the least understood sense, according to Kenneth Johnson, former Professor of Neuroscience at Hopkins' Krieger Mind/Brain Institute. The fingertips, lips, and tongue are the most pain-sensitive sites on the body and report very specific information quickly. Our hands contain about a hundred thousand nerves of at least 20 different kinds, 12 of which report various touch sensations. The rapidity with which the neurons fire determines the intensity of the pain that is experienced. Myelinated fibers conduct faster messages, and those from unmyelinated neurons travel more slowly. Pain messages are transmitted from the left side of the body to the right side of the brain and vice versa. Other sites of pain can be more difficult to pinpoint; the brain, for example, has no pain receptors. The most common types of pain are referred to using the following terms:

- Acute—from a recent injury or trauma.
- Chronic—regardless of the source of the pain, the sensation lingers beyond the initial trigger.
- Neuropathic—when the nervous system is damaged or functioning incorrectly, the pain signals are often stabbing, burning, or tingling, often associated with Heat and Blood stasis.
- Nociceptive—specialized sensory nerve fibers called nociceptors are located in the skin, musculature, joints, and some organs, and transmit pain signals to the brain.
- Radicular—leg pain which radiates from the back and hips along the spinal nerve root. This pain is often sharp and accompanied by numbness, weakness, and paresthesia. Associated with Deficiency, Dampness, Stasis, and Stagnation.
- Referral pain—when pain is perceived in an area other than the part of the body that experiences pathology. For example, gallbladder pain can be experienced in the right shoulder. Heart pain can be felt down the arm, shoulder, or back, as spinal segments share nerve pathways, and the brain can't tell them apart.
- Somatic pain—pain from the skin, subcutaneous tissues, muscles, and joints.
- Visceral pain—vague and diffuse pressure-type pain caused by damage or inflammation to the internal organs, which have few pain receptors; the sensation is often conveyed to other parts of the body.

Chinese medicine, of course, considers all pain to be due to hindered flow. Sometimes our greatest anguish has psychogenic origins, and if we haven't been taught how to be present with the source of our discomfort, it can manifest somatically. The free circulation of Qi and Blood can be impaired in order to limit movement so we will attend to the obstruction and/or protect the injured area so we don't cause further damage. While the inciting event of damaged tissues occurs locally, pain is registered in the mind, which then projects sensations onto the body to protect itself. When the Qi is obstructed, the pain is experienced as cramps or distension. When due to Cold, pain is experienced as severe and tight. The area may be cold to the touch, be worse in cold, and circulation is often impaired. When due to Dampness, the area is experienced as heavy, and when Blood stasis is the culprit, the sensation is stabbing and boring, fixed in location, and the area may become darker in color and might be associated with varicosities. Wind will cause the pain to move throughout the body, come on chaotically, be associated with twitching or spasms, and perhaps involve itching.

Chinese herbs which have analgesic effects include Dan Shen, Dang Gui, Du Duo, Du Zhong, Fang Feng, Gan Cao, Gan Jiang, Gui Zhi, Ling Zhi, Long Kui, Mu Dan Pi, Mu Tong, Nou Xi, Qing Hao, Qin Jiao, Ren Shen, Sheng Ma, Suan Zao Ren, Tian Nan Xing, Wu Zhu Yu, Xi Xin, Xiang Fu, Xian He Cao, Yi Ren, Zhi Zi.

Herbs with anti-inflammatory properties include Chai Hu, Che Qian Cao, Da Qing Ye, Dan Pi, Dan Shen, Dang Gui, Du Hou, Du Zhong, Fang Feng, Fu Zi Gan Cao, Gan Jiang, Ge Gen, Huang Qin, Jin Yin Hua, Lai Fu Zi, Lian Qiao, Long Dan Cao, Long Kui, Ma Huang, Mu Tong, Nou Xi, Pu Huang, Qin Jiao, Qin Pi, Ren Shen, Sheng Ma, Shu Di, Shui Niu Jiao, Xi Xian Cao, Xi Xin, Xian He Cao, Xiang Fu, Xuan Shen, Yin Yang Huo, Yu Xing Cao.

On the way from acute to chronic, three primary stages of injury have been defined:

- The immediate effects after the trauma, usually three to five days unless the injury is severe. Characterized by swelling, redness, pain, and difficulty mobilizing, this stage represents Heat and Blood stagnation, so our treatment principles will be to clear Heat and move Blood. Take caution applying ice, as this can cause more Stasis and perhaps bring pathology into Latency where it may become chronic. Herbs like San Qi or Yunnan Baiyao can be used to stop bleeding without causing Stasis. Die Da Wan or Fu Yuan Huo Cue Tang are great Blood movers as well. You may use bleeding with cupping, and/or bleed the Jing Well points.

- During the transitional stage, we need to evaluate where the pathogenic factor is and where it's going. While we may be clearing Heat, we may also need to warm the channels. What channel is affected? To which stage has it progressed?
- If the trauma becomes chronic, the pathogenic factor has sunken in, perhaps because of Cold or Dampness. We need to move Qi and Blood while warming the channels. We might consider formulations like Du Huo Ji Sheng Tang and Juan Bi Tang to address Wind Damp Bi syndrome.

Treatment may include working with the sinew channels, opening the involved channel, and using the Xi Cleft points, Jing Well points, Ashi points, and local and distant points. The six stages through which pathogens progress correspond to six levels of movement:

- Leg Tai Yang—associated with forward and extension movements that propel us forward, Leg Tai Yang follows the UB channel, which is often weakened with excessive sitting for long periods of time. Any type of back pain, along with tension and occipital headaches, is a common Leg Tai Yang pattern. UB 60 and UB 63 are often included in treatments.
- Leg Shao Yang—associated with rotation, pivoting, side-to-side motion, and asymmetrical tilting. Include GB 34, GB 21, and/or GB 30.
- Leg Yang Ming—associated with stopping, bracing, bearing weight; opposes Leg Tai Yang forward movement through bracing the anterior muscles that correspond to the Stomach channel (rectus abdominus), and includes urogenital and bowel involvement. St 36, St 37, and St 39 are often helpful.
- Arm Tai Yang—involves extension of the arm and shoulder. GB 12 and SI 3 are useful.
- Arm Shao Yang—rotation of the arm, goes to the tongue and neck. SJ 3, SJ 6, SJ 7.
- Arm Yang Ming—lateral extension, LI 7 and LI 10 help.

The Yin levels of movement are:

- Tai Yin involves flexion movement inward.
- Shao Yin includes rotation in flexion, and protecting the Heart.
- The Jue Yin stage is characterized by the absence of movement.

While we might be called on to facilitate the healing of and reduce pain in the case of acute injuries, our services are most often utilized when one experiences ongoing, chronic pain, especially back pain. Studies have shown that between a quarter and three-quarters of the adult population experiences back pain, which accounts for almost 40 percent of all reported pain conditions for which patients seek relief. Chronic back pain corresponds with Leg Tai Yang patterns, which are most often associated with a history of excess forward movement. The way we drive ourselves to accomplish, physically, mentally, and emotionally, contributes to the development of Tai Yang patterns. When we continually attempt to fuel ourselves through worldly acquisitions or accomplishments, our Kidneys become depleted. While Foot Tai Yang is abundant in early life, it often lacks the foundational power necessary to take us into our later years, when our source of strength should shift from Kidney Jing dominance to the Shen as it lifts us to walk more lightly on our journey toward ascension.

According to John Sarno (1999), in *Mind Over Back Pain*, rarely is back pain purely structural. Conditions such as herniated discs, spondylolisthesis, scoliosis, and pinched nerves are usually misdiagnoses. Abnormalities which are strictly structural are just as likely to be asymptomatic than to cause pain. The pain associated with these types of presentations more commonly results from a condition he refers to as tension myositis syndrome where ongoing tension, the type often experienced by the chronic psycho-emotional holding patterns in the posturing of Type A personalities, constricts blood vessels and restricts circulation in the musculature. When this type of pain becomes chronic or even episodic, the fear of further injury, another spasm, spinal degeneration, disc herniation, or potential disability further contracts the musculature, impeding movement. It's a vicious cycle that rarely is resolved through conventional measures like surgery or medication.

Sometimes surgery relieves the pain, which Sarno believes is largely due to the placebo effect. Surgery is elected when a condition is quite severe, and it is believed that cutting directly into the area to repair tissues or remove excess debris will treat the source. Much of the healing happens because the patient is required to become immobilized after the surgical procedure. Orthopedic surgery is often attempted even when there is no structural reason, but rarely is it 100 percent effective in relieving chronic back pain, and many patients end up in pain clinics for ongoing injections and narcotic administration after "failed" back surgeries.

Biopsies from the muscles of patients with chronic back pain display changes in muscle cells indicative of oxygen deprivation. Unresolved conflict produces tension, which obstructs free flow. That which is unconsciously repressed or consciously suppressed often resurfaces as the person's attempts to put the discomfort out of their mind have failed. Attempting to bypass uncomfortable feelings by ignoring them or focusing only on the positive may relegate them to the unconscious, but still produces subclinical anxiety and generates tension, which obstructs the free flow of Qi and Blood, resulting in pain.

If the effects of muscular tension deplete the flow of Qi and Blood, and exhaust the Kidneys and Liver, which govern the tendons, we are left with brittle musculature, deprived of warmth. Dampness settles in to protect, and Wind produces micro spasms. If we evaluate the functions of Du Huo Ji Sheng Tang, it treats precisely that dynamic by tonifying the Kidneys and Liver, Qi, and Blood, and also expelling Wind, Damp, and Cold.

The intense sensations of ongoing pain can lock one into a heightened perception of physical sensations. The resulting contraction and resistance to pain usually produce more suffering than the actual pain sensations themselves. The corporeal soul, Po, is our instinctual animal body, and we all have witnessed animals in pain. While they might writhe and yelp to escape intensely painful sensations, they do not continue to suffer by remembering and resisting the pain signals as humans do. This is one of the ways that the drug ketamine works. Ketamine is a dissociative anesthetic which does nothing for injuries to the tissues or pain signals per se; instead it detaches the patient from the bodily sensations and makes them "forget" the pain and become unresponsive to stimuli. Sometimes producing hallucinations and "out of body" experiences, it disassociates the Hun from the Po. While this might produce fun recreational effects in immature users, this is never an effect we want to maintain if we are going for higher states of health and wellness. When we keep our attention directly in the center of the pain, it can not only reveal the source of the pain, but can also become a portal to what lies beyond the physical without dissociating from it. The Po become our allies when united with the Hun.

Marta, usually quite fit and healthy, was in her late fifties when she experienced intense back pain which came on not long after a prolonged and intense family drama. She said she always had a "weak back," as did everyone in her family. After being chastised for going against some deep-seated familial beliefs and behavioral rules, she was cut off from holiday gatherings. Feeling depressed and traumatized, she desperately needed a break from the troubling dynamic, so she went on a shopping trip with some girlfriends. In the fitting room of a clothing store, with no warning at all, her low back seized with excruciating pain, after which she couldn't stand up straight or walk. Her friends helped her back into her clothes and into the car and urged her to take anti-inflammatories, muscle relaxants, and to apply ice to her back, which she resisted. While it hurt immensely, she knew she hadn't injured anything, that this was a psychological manifestation. She remained present to her experience of pain while she applied heat, took an epsom salt bath, got a massage, and had acupuncture to harmonize the Liver and Spleen and open up the spine. The pressure on her paraspinal musculature was excruciating and felt like heavy leaden bands that didn't even belong to her body.

With this type of pain presentation, I encourage patients to bring their attention to the area where pain is registering and be fully present with it. What qualities does it exhibit? Does it have a particular color, texture, or temperature? Pain speaks a somatic language of the Po, purely sensory. While they can ask themselves what pressure is being manifested or what stressful emotion is being suppressed or has been repressed, rarely do the Po speak through logical, therapeutic storylines. But as the Po communicate with the Hun, the origin of the pain often reveals itself.

Marta was supported to stay with her sensations, which intensified and spread throughout her musculature—down her legs, up her back, and into her shoulders and neck. She remained present with the pain until it crescendoed. She experienced it as a blackish green, heavy tar-like substance, cold and sluggish, which was *holding her back*—figuratively and literally. In that moment, she realized that her muscles and tendons were releasing the weight of a burden to try to please her family that she had been carrying her whole life. And in that realization, it began to subside until within a few minutes it was over. The experience felt as if her body let go of her need to please along with the pain, and the depressed mood left with it.

True healing can be quite radical. It doesn't view the body through a reductionist lens that merely tries to alleviate the symptoms or patch up the most broken parts. It understands that symptoms are indicators, and if we follow the manifestation back to the source, we find the trigger that set off the myriad displays of psychic and physical confusion. We are restored. Marta's acute back spasm was caused by the chronic anguish of a lifetime of unhealthy family dynamics, tucked deeply away in the subconscious, that caused her to feel that she was never enough and held her back from living fully. The experience was life changing for her, and she said she was literally a different person afterwards. The only emotion left was gratitude for what the pain had revealed to her.

Blood stasis

Blood oxygenates nerves, and good blood flow is essential to keep their messages flowing freely. When an area becomes stagnant and blood flow diminishes, pain can indicate toxic build-up of waste products in the tissues, deoxygenation, and the stabbing pain associated with Blood stasis. Static Blood can also be associated with psychic stasis, where one's Heart and Pericardium are bound by protective holding patterns. Invigorating the Heart Blood to resolve old identity structures can transfigure the being and leave the spirit in an intoxicated state of ecstatic wonder.

Ecstasy has been defined as a state of mind where there is no stasis. In fact, the word was originally used by 17th-century mystics to describe a rapturous state where the soul could stand outside one's physicality and contemplate divine states of consciousness. These higher states of mind can be accessed through hallucinogenic drugs that strongly invigorate the Heart Blood to produce temporary blissful states, which will pass unless one integrates the expansive states of Shen and incorporates them into the ability to rewire the entire body-mind structure. We can only assume that these experiences are accompanied by the release of pineal and pituitary hormones.

Endorphins

One of the main ways in which acupuncture provides relief is by interrupting the transmission of pain signals to the brain, while simultaneously facilitating the release of endorphins. Endorphins are endogenous morphine-like peptide hormones produced primarily by the pituitary gland in response to pain or stress. They make us feel good, and even have the power to transform painful sensations into euphoric states. There are many types of endorphins, some of which are released during injury, torment, or childbirth; others might be stimulated by sex, the release of tears, or even by ultraviolet light hitting the skin. Belonging to the domain of Metal, endorphins blanket the harsh sensations of the world and can draw us inward, where they disable the warning signals associated with pain, replacing them with euphoric neuropeptides that can cloud the orifices of the Heart while we are provided relief.

A great example of this process is when a woman is in the process of giving birth. As her cervix opens, waves of intensity are sent coursing through her system, which the mind can interpret as extremely painful, when resisted, and are usually accompanied by thoughts like *This hurts too much. I can't do it!* Should she be able to lean into the heightened sensations of the birthing process, the same experience can become fiercely orgasmic. If she is not utilizing exogenous epidural or opioid pain medication to cover up the pain, she can remain alert and able to respond to her emerging child, while her system will be flooded with endogenous endorphins, producing euphoric states of consciousness through labor and delivery.

Pain relievers

Now let's look at what happens when we take a drug to block the perception of pain. Pharmaceuticals don't restore free flow, they mute physiologic responses to pain. Quelling the sensation of pain is considered suppressive in nature, as we are in a state of resistance to the experience of pain we are having. Any suppressive process like Cold or Dampness can stagnate the flow of Qi, which can then give rise to depressive Heat. Analgesics produce a state of Cold in the Liver, whose job is to keep our Qi flowing freely. The very act of masking the pain hinders the Liver's Qi mechanism. It's much like closing our eyes when we are afraid to look at something. It doesn't go away, but we can pretend it isn't there.

When working with someone on pain relievers, their tongue and pulse will reveal the pharmaceutical's specific effects on their Qi and Blood. The Liver pulse will often be wiry, not just from the pain, but because of the Liver constraint caused by the analgesic. Here we need to relax the Liver and protect the Stomach and Spleen. In addition to treating their pain pattern, we may also have to calm the Shen, move the Qi and Blood, and resolve any stagnation the medicine may have induced.

Long-term use of analgesics can affect Yang Ming, and can cause the Liver to overact on the Spleen and Stomach. They can cause the imbalance to move further down and in, so we need to protect the Yang Ming, and because analgesics have an effect on the production of Qi and Blood, we need to be aware of their effect on Tai Yin levels. Pain relievers have also been found to inhibit the electron chain transport involved in generating the electrochemical gradient that drives ATP synthesis, greatly stagnating the Qi mechanism.

Analgesics can cause bleeding and water retention, especially in the Stomach. Chai Hu formulas can regulate descension of Stomach with Zhi Shi, Bai Shao, and Gan Cao, and protect the Stomach from bleeding. Wu Wei Zi and Dang Gui can also help protect the Liver.

Non-steroidal anti-inflammatory drugs (NSAIDs)

- Celecoxib (Celebrex)
- Diclofenac (Cataflam, Voltaren, Arthrose)

- Diflunisal (Dolobid), etodolac (Lodine)
- Fenoprofen (Nalfon), flurbiprofen (Ansaid)
- Ibuprofen (Motrin, Tab-Prüfen)
- Indomethacin (Indocin)
- Ketoprofen (Oruvail)
- Ketorolac (Toradol)
- Mefenamic acid (Ponstel)
- Meloxicam (Mobic)
- Nabumetone (Related)
- Naproxen (Naprosyn, Anaprox, Naprelan, Naprapac)
- Oxaprozin (Daypro)
- Piroxicam (Feldene)
- Sulindac (Clinoril)
- Tolmetin (Tolectin)

Damaged tissues release prostaglandins, a group of pro-inflammatory lipids that initiate local Wei Qi responses. Prostaglandins are arachidonic acid metabolites, which modulate inflammation, body temperature, pain transmission, and platelet aggregation, as well as being essential in causing ovulation and uterine contractions during menses and labor. They are released on demand, and rapidly degrade. When one is hurt, prostaglandins dilate local blood vessels so that more blood flow arrives to the injured area. Fluid is also diverted to the area, causing swelling. As immune mediators arrive, the area becomes red, hot, swollen, and inflamed. Cyclooxygenase (Cox) 1 and 2 are enzymes that catalyze the production of prostaglandins. Cox-1 is present throughout the body tissues; it maintains the mucosal lining of the stomach and small intestines, and impacts platelets and the kidneys. Cox-2 is involved with local inflammatory reactions. Most NSAIDs block both of these enzymes, inhibiting the Yang effects of prostaglandins, thereby reducing local Wei Qi inflammatory reactions, and Wei Qi's function in protecting the gut. NSAIDs reduce blood flow to the kidneys, causing the build-up of fluid which increases blood pressure. This process can become toxic to and damage the kidneys. NSAIDs also tend to slow the time it takes for the blood to clot. Like herbs that Cool and Invigorate the Blood, they can also damage Spleen and Kidney Yang. When Yang is impaired, so is its ability to move the Blood, potentially resulting in thrombotic episodes. Like aspirin, NSAIDs can induce sweating by distorting Wei Qi's role in opening and closing the pores. And because NSAIDs are metabolized in the Liver, their use can result in Liver Qi stagnation. And Qi stagnation can always give rise to depressive Heat.

Aspirin—acetylsalicylic acid (ASA)

- Ascriptin, Aspirate, Bayer, Bufferin, Easprin, Ecotrin, Ecpirin, Entercote, Excedrin, Genacote, Halfprin, Ninoprin, Norwich

Willow and meadowsweet grow along the banks of rivers and marshy areas. Their ability to thrive in damp environments endowed them with properties that could relieve joint pain, recognized by the ancient Egyptians, Assyrians, Chinese, Romans, and Native American civilizations for thousands of years. Meadowsweet was a sacred herb of the Celts, and in the late 1700s a British preacher found that willow bark could consistently lower fevers. In the mid 1800s, a German professor figured out the chemical structure of salicylic acid which was derived from the bark of the willow tree. It tasted nasty and irritated the stomach, but by the turn of the century a chemist at Bayer & Co., Felix Hoffmann, manipulated the chemical makeup until he was able to produce a more stable compound, acetylsalicylic acid. In 1899, aspirin was registered as the first synthetically derived pharmaceutical drug, which birthed the entire pharmaceutical industry. In the mid-1900s, aspirin was also found to inhibit platelet aggregation, and its list of effects has grown.

Aspirin was the first NSAID, and it reduces inflammation, relieves pain, lowers temperatures of febrile patients, has an antifungal effect, reduces cholesterol crystal expansion, and prevents platelet aggregation. Platelets belong to the Spleen's ability to bank the Blood. They are also primary carriers of serotonin, which helps constrict vessels and clumps platelets together to form blood clots. The side effects of aspirin use include increased bleeding, easy bruisability, decreased urine output, gastrointestinal upset, and ulcers. Prostaglandins have Yang effects that Heat the Blood, while their effect in the gut regulates fluid transfer, inhibits the secretion of the very Yang hydrochloric acid, alters mucosal blood flow, and stimulates Yin mucus and bicarbonate secretion. Thus, when you block Cox, prostaglandins are inhibited. This then reverses the above effects, reducing Yang effects of Heat in the periphery, while increasing the invigorating effects of Yang in the gut, drying Stomach Yin, resulting in irritation and potential damage to the stomach lining by hydrochloric acid. As pathogenic factors proceed from the external to the internal, the Yang Qi may move into the chest as in Shao Yang conditions. Aspirin can force the Qi into the substernal region, where it can invade the Stomach and Spleen, resulting in Yang Ming Heat, which can give rise to gastric bleeding. The stagnancy in the chest can create a scenario where Si Ni San could be used to harmonize Shao Yang. Herbs that generate fluids in the Stomach at the Shao Yang stage, like Zhi Mu, can also be used to protect the Stomach and clear Heat. Those taking aspirin tend to have wiry pulses due to constraint in the Liver.

We can see then that aspirin's effects are mostly suppressive and stagnating in nature but it does have dispersing effects. ASA clears Heat, invigorates Blood, and discourages Damp Phlegm, while it also hinders the Spleen in banking the Blood. It can dry out Stomach Yin, which can result in a heating effect in the gut, potentially giving rise to bleeding of the gums or ulcers. Aspirin might be a good choice for addressing acute conditions of Damp Bi, but is not considered effective long term. The effects on the Stomach are going to be more severe in patients who are deficient in Stomach Yin. The state of Liver Blood and Qi will also be impacted by aspirin's cooling, drying effects. Liver toxicity may result from stagnated Liver Heat. The pulse will often be wiry, or choppy in the left Guan position. Further, any drug which strongly invigorates the Blood can exhaust Kidney Yang. Aspirin can also reduce vitamin E and folic acid levels, and leach zinc out of the bones.

Ibuprofen

- Addaprin, Advil, AG Profen, Bufen, Genpril, Haltran, Ibu, Ibuprohm, Ibu-Tab, I-Prin, Midol, Motrin, Nuprin, Proprinal, Q-Profen

Ibuprofen is a non-steroidal anti-inflammatory drug that prevents prostaglandin synthesis by non-selectively inhibiting Cyclooxygenase 1 and 2. Because it has a relatively quick onset and is short acting, it must be re-administered every four to six hours and is thus more helpful for acute conditions.

Taking ibuprofen can result in bleeding, loss of iron, increases in sodium, and edema. Like aspirin, it relieves pain and inflammation and reduces fever, but with fewer GI side effects, and does not reduce platelet aggregation or cholesterol crystal expansion. Thus, ibuprofen clears Heat, with less of an effect of invigorating Blood or resolving Dampness. The cooling effect can impair the dynamics of the Spleen and Stomach, and large doses over time can result in liver failure, as the Liver overacts on the Spleen.

Cox-1 selective NSAIDs

- Ketorolac (Acular)
- Flurbiprofen (Ocufen)
- Ketoprofen (Generic)
- Indomethacin (Indocin)
- Tolmetin (Generic)
- Piroxicam (Feline)
- Meclofenamate (Generic)
- Naproxen (Aleve, Naproxyn)

In addition to protecting the mucosal lining of the gut, Cox-1 enzymes encourage blood to clot and arteries to constrict. Thus, NSAIDs that block Cox-1 can produce the opposite effects, causing vasodilation, thinning the blood, and drying out of Stomach Yin. Naproxen has a longer therapeutic duration, so only needs to be taken twice per day and is thus more appropriate for chronic conditions. Being more Cox-1 selective, while naproxen doesn't increase the risk for thrombotic events, this must be weighed against its increased risk for causing gastrointestinal symptoms.

Cox-2 selective NSAIDs

- Sulindac (Clinoril)
- Diclofenac (Cambia)
- Celecoxib (Celebrex)
- Meloxicam (Mobic)
- Etodolac (Generic)

Cox-2 inhibitors pinpoint inflammation and have fewer GI side effects, because Cox-2 doesn't impact the lining of the gut. This reduces Heat, but if only Cox-2 is blocked, it causes an imbalance in prostacyclin, leaving Cox-1 unchecked. This encourages the formation of clots and vasoconstriction, increasing the potential risk for heart attacks or strokes. Cox-2 inhibitors clear Heat, yet when Yang is hindered from moving the Blood, it can leave Blood stasis in its wake.

Acetaminophen (Tylenol)

Acetaminophen is not an NSAID. It has both analgesic and antipyretic actions, but no anti-inflammatory properties, so does not reduce swelling, nor does it have anti-thrombotic effects. It also produces less GI irritation, so is prescribed more often when minor aches and pains or fever are present. It has less potential for kidney toxicity, but can cause severe liver damage, especially in those who have liver disease or drink much alcohol. The use of Tylenol has been implicated as one of the major causes of liver failure requiring liver transplants. Side effects include skin rash, itching, nausea, vomiting, and constipation. While the exact mechanism is unknown, Tylenol seems to act by increasing the nervous system's pain threshold; it impacts the ability of the hypothalamus to regulate body temperature, but has little effect on the Wei Qi. Tylenol impacts the Liver, Spleen, and Stomach, and digesting carbohydrates can interfere with its action. It should be taken with protein. Broccoli and cabbage also impact Tylenol's effects. Muting the nervous system and decreasing body temperature are Cold effects, which can strongly stagnate the Liver. This can produce depressive Heat, counterflow side effects, and Heat-type allergic reactions in those prone to Heat or whose Yang may already have been unrooted.

Corticosteroids

Before we talk about muting the adrenal response, let's discuss the physio-logic functions of the adrenal hormones, the reflection of how Kidney Yin and Yang are utilized. The adrenal glands provide the "spark plugs" to initiate energy production, including the quick Yang response of Wei Qi. The San Jiao mechanism helps maintain homeostasis between water balance, reproductive hormones, and the fight/flight response. Fear and anxiety cause stress hormones to induce the hyper-arousal of the primitive nervous system, which unroots Kidney Yang from its source, making it flare upward. This upward movement is antagonistic to the reproductive hormones.

In response to short-term stressors, nerve cells in the brain act on the sympathetic nervous system in the spinal cord to directly stimulate the adrenal medulla (the Yin core of the adrenal gland) to release epinephrine and norepinephrine, Yang hormones that activate the heart to become alert to danger. This surge in Kidney Yang increases metabolic rate, oxygen consumption, and heat production, while breaking glycogen down to glucose, thereby elevating blood glucose levels. It also increases blood pressure and breathing rate, and makes us more alert by diverting blood flow away from the digestive, kidney, and reproductive functions, and sending it to the brain, eyes, and large muscle groups instead.

This type of Yang stimulation can burn us out as we rely on the spark plugs for energy production, rather than the slow release of Kidney Qi. In response, the upper control centers sense the excess Yang and cause the pituitary gland to release adrenocorticotropic hormone, which then acts on the adrenal gland to compensate by releasing corticosteroids so we don't burn out our essence. Cortisol, the Yin within the Yang cortex of the adrenal gland, is then released to Dampen the Heat response; it also acts on the Liver to raise blood glucose levels and mobilize glucose stores for long-term stress, which has a Yin or Dampening effect on the body.

When Wei Qi is diverted to address tissue damage, its immune activating Yang effects rush to the area to patch up the repair, resulting in the uncomfortable effects of Heat, inflammation, and swelling. Cortisol can be used to mute these immune system responses.

Glucocorticoids

- Cortisone, hydrocortisone, prednisone, prednisolone, methylprednisolone, dexamethasone

Cortisone and its synthetic derivatives are used to control pain, inflammation, and overactive allergic or immune responses, by inhibiting Kidney Yang's contribution to Wei Qi. Side effects include increased breakdown of muscle, skin, lymph, adipose, and connective tissue, causing thinning of the skin, easy bruisability, muscle wasting, agitation, insomnia, depression, hyperglycemia, weight gain as well as edema, puffy face, hypertension from fluid retention, osteoporosis, cataracts, and glaucoma. These effects can be attributed to an unrooted Ming Men Fire, disruption of San Jiao's ability to maintain the waterways, and disruption of the Heart-Kidney axis. Impaired Kidney Yang can no longer support the Spleen Qi in its holding or transformation roles, resulting in Damp accumulation and eventually Phlegm. As ongoing cortisol administration continues to mute Kidney Yang, the suppressed immune system increases susceptibility to other infectious processes. If prescribed in high doses or for prolonged periods of time, it can cause the adrenal gland to cease production of its own glucocorticoids, eventually leading to cortical atrophy. Our treatments can help by tonifying and anchoring the Kidneys and Spleen, and resolving Dampness.

Tolerance and addiction can develop as well. Those on steroids for significant periods of time can experience a debilitating condition when they stop the glucocorticoids, known as steroid withdrawal syndrome, characterized by an exacerbation of the original symptoms for which the corticosteroids were prescribed. In addition, patients experience fatigue, irritability, depression, shaking, loss of appetite, nausea, aches, pain, lightheadedness, and insomnia. This is one of the reasons dosages are slowly tapered down instead of abruptly ceased. The Kidneys and Spleen energies, which have been muted, take some time to restore normal function.

When topical steroids are withdrawn for skin conditions, skin irritation can come back with a vengeance. Burning, weeping, oozing, cracking, peeling, itching, and painful skin can accompany this scenario and can last up to eight weeks. This is a type of rebound phenomena where, since the underlying causative issues were never addressed, the Dampness caused by the steroids only temporarily kept symptoms at bay. This creates an environment where Dampness traps Heat pathogens, which then emerge all at once when the steroids are withdrawn.

GABA analogue: gabapentin (Neurontin, Gralise, Neuraptine, Horizant)

The anticonvulsant/antiepileptic drug gabapentin is prescribed to treat seizures and address neuropathic pain, including diabetic neuropathy, post-herpetic neuralgia, and central neuropathic pain. Glutamate is an amino acid that acts as an excitatory Yang neurotransmitter in the nervous system, whereas GABA has a Yin or inhibitory effect. GABA analogues reduce the excitability of nerve cells by enhancing GABA activity and inhibiting an enzyme in glutamate synthesis, and are also prescribed to address the symptoms of restless leg syndrome, as well as some anxiety and panic disorders. The action of gabapentin, in part, is understood to inhibit high-voltage dependent calcium channels involved in the transmission of nerve impulses. GABA's Yin effect induces states of relaxation which calm the Shen. Gabapentin decreases excessive Heart Yang stimulation, with a cooling and anchoring effect that can stagnate the Qi to slow down neural stimulation and settle excessive Yang. Side effects include fatigue, peripheral edema, low libido, and dizziness. Patients with Heart Fire often do very well on this medication, but those with deficient Heart Yang will be likely to experience more side effects. Those with underlying Heart deficiencies may be more prone to gabapentin's tendency to cause mood and behavioral changes like depression, anxiety, and thoughts of suicide.

Antispasmodic skeletal muscle relaxants (SMR)

- Carisoprodol (Soma)
- Chlorzoxazone (Parafòn Ferte, Lorzone)
- Cyclobenzaprine (Fexmid, Flexeril, Amrix)
- Metaxalone (Skelaxin, Metaxall)
- Methocarbamol (Robaxin)
- Orphenadrine (Norflex)
- Tizanidine (Zanaflex)

Muscle relaxants do not directly exert their effects on the muscles. These centrally acting muscle relaxants depress the central nervous system in order to interrupt the nerve signals being received by the brain. While not more effective than NSAIDs or acetaminophen in providing pain relief, their side effects include headache, dizziness, drowsiness, sedation, lowered blood pressure, dry mouth, nervousness, and confusion. Some, like carisoprodol, cyclobenzaprine, and tizanidine, may be habit forming as they can cause a relaxing, euphoric state, and are often overused, giving rise to addiction, overdose, and death. Their effects cool the Liver and suppress Liver Yang to reduce the Wind which is responsible for causing muscle spasms. If Liver Yang is hyperactive, the therapeutic effect might be noticeable. Those with Liver Qi stagnation or Cold in the Liver, however, will probably experience more negative than therapeutic effects.

Opioids

- Morphine (Apokyn, Kadian, Avinza, MS-Contin)
- Hydrocodone (Vicodin)
- Oxycodone (Oxycontin, Percocet)
- Oxymorphone (Opana)
- Codeine, fentanyl (Actiq, Duragesic, Fentora, Lazanda, Subsys)
- Sufentanyl, hydromorphone (Dilauded)
- Tapentadol (Nucynta)
- Tramadol (Ultram)
- Methadone (Dolophine, Methadose)

Endogenous endorphins exert their actions on opioid receptors in the brain, spinal cord, and peripheral nociceptors, the system responsible for our ability to feel. In the central nervous system, there are three types of opioid receptors: mu, delta, and kappa. Opioid receptors are also present in the gastrointestinal autonomic nervous system. They are used to depress the central nervous system, reduce the perception of pain, induce euphoria, and promote sleep. Opioids are a class of drugs derived from the resin released by the poppy plant when its surface is injured. Like opium, they mimic the actions of endorphins, enkephalins (which regulate pain sensations), and dynorphins (involved in the regulation of pain, moods, and addiction) by binding to all three opioid receptors. Opioid agonists mute the sensation of pain by binding to the mu receptor within the central and peripheral nervous system, and are often used for anesthesia. They also reduce coughing and intestinal motility, and may lead to side effects such as constipation, cholestasis, nausea, vomiting, dry mouth, sleepiness, lethargy, dizziness, confusion, psychomotor impairment, slurred speech, pupillary constriction or dilation, depression, itching, sweating, and increased pain sensitivity.

Opium was initially used medicinally in China as the tonifying and astringing herb Ying Su Ke, the husk of the poppy plant. Li Shi Zhen categorized its effects as being able to treat pain, cough, and diarrhea. Opioids have a stabilizing effect in the Lower Jiao, as they bind the Kidneys and Intestines, astringing the bowels, vaginal discharge, and sperm leakage. Li Shi Zhen also highlighted opium's ability to delay ejaculation by retaining the male essence, thus enhancing virility. In the 1400s, opium became more popular as a recreational drug because of its euphoric and aphrodisiac effects, giving rise to opium dens centuries later. A morphine derivative, diacetylmorphine (heroin) was isolated in the late 1800s by a German scientist. Almost a hundred years later, the Bayer Company began to produce heroin commercially, which was marketed for rheumatism, tuberculosis, bronchitis, asthma, as well as many other disorders, and the treatment of codeine and morphine addiction. Today, narcotics like morphine are used to provide relief from pain during and after surgery, cancer, end-of-life care, and almost any other condition where the patient experiences moderate to severe pain.

The term narcotic derives from the Greek term *narco*, which means to make numb. Their sedating effect on the mind is caused by astringing the Lungs and binding Lung Yin, which temporarily mutes the Po's sensations. Since Metal controls Wood, the strong astringing effect on the Lung can overact on the Liver Luo, producing an aphrodisiac effect, although opioids also deplete testosterone levels. The Po are closely related to the autonomic nervous system, the sensory receptors, especially the primitive touch responses of the skin, and the interior sense receptors of the visceral organs. The Hun are overly aroused, and the sedated Po are no longer able to communicate with the Hun, and while the body's sensations are muted, the unrooted Hun can temporarily enchant the Heart-Mind. This causes a separation between the Hun and the Po, and when the initial euphoric effect is over and the narcotic is withdrawn, the opposite effect is produced as the Po arouse, agitating the nervous system, leaving one in a state of extreme unrest and hypersensitivity. The Liver may become damaged, the Hun lose their grounding, and Blood stasis in the Liver may ensue, which also traumatizes the Pericardium. Patients on narcotics, especially long term, may become tormented by extreme unease, apathy, slowed cognition, and impaired mental functioning, and they may crave the euphoric state again.

Tolerance develops, requiring more of the drug for the same effect, and as the Hun and Po remain separated, the psyche continues in states of anguish, which gives rise to the drug's highly addictive tendency. This cycle can be extremely difficult to break, and manifests as a type of possession that is nearly impossible to escape from without intervention. It is estimated that about 16 million people worldwide suffer from opioid use disorder and in 2020 the US Congress Joint Economic Committee reported that the opioid epidemic cost the United States almost 1.5 trillion dollars. Narcotic prescriptions are not to be taken lightly (JEC, n.d.).

Opioid withdrawal syndrome can occur even after small amounts of pharmaceuticals are given. After larger doses for longer periods of time, withdrawal can be extremely dangerous, and potentially fatal, as Yin and Yang veer toward extreme separation. When one is dependent on the drug and stops abruptly, withdrawal syndrome is characterized by effects that are opposite to the drug's use: dysphoria, anxiety, craving, restlessness, muscle aches, diaphoresis, tachycardia, vomiting, and leakage from most other orifices, which can result in dehydration. Narcotic overdose can cause respiratory failure for which opioid antagonists like naloxone are administered to interrupt the narcotic effects.

Morphine is the most common pharmaceutical given during end-of-life care to address discomfort, pain, and breathing difficulties. While nobody would argue this is a kindness, the complexity of how the soul relinquishes its hold on life so it can move on can be impaired by narcotic administration—a topic which is covered more extensively in the Conclusion at the end of this book.

Helping to overcome addiction and cravings

Depending on patients' underlying patterns of imbalance and the effects of the drug, acupuncture can help wean a person off their medication, but isn't considered a stand-alone therapy without medical supervision, psychotherapy, and some type of support program. While removing the need for the drug will be the immediate focus, underlying causative factors must be addressed. Not everyone who takes narcotics will become addicted, nor will everyone who drinks alcohol become an alcoholic. Addictive personalities meet some of the criteria of Shen disturbances, and according to Carl Jung, those who become addicted to spirits often have a severe spiritual longing that only "spirits" can satiate.

The particular effects of each mind-altering substance vary as well. Alcohol, for example, produces Damp Heat in the Liver. Tetrahydrocannabinol (THC) causes Yang stimulation to the Hun and may result in excess Liver Yang scenarios, or cause the Liver to overact on the Spleen, which weakens its attention capacity and may lead to Dampness. Cannabidiol (CBD) nourishes Liver Yin and Blood and can anchor the Hun; and psychedelics may overstimulate the Hun and Shen at the Blood level. Continued use can lead to rebound Blood stasis.

Dependency, cravings, and addiction cause alterations in the brain, especially in the ventral striatum that initiates the craving, the insula that acts on it, and the prefrontal cortex which controls the emotions. These correspond to the Zang organs of the Kidney, Liver, and Heart, and the fibers that connect them all belong to the Spleen. Psychologically, deficient Kidney energies can be associated with insecurities, lack of self-worth, and self-esteem, resulting in a feeling of emptiness. A person then longs for a substance to make them feel better, which equates with the Liver's tendency to reach for higher states, causing the Hun to rise. If the Liver Blood is insufficient to keep up with the external reaching for more, it can cause Stagnation and Heat, which rise up to disturb the Heart. The Qi becomes loose, the Shen no longer have a still and tranquil home, and the spirits scatter, and can no longer keep the Hun in check. And, of course, extreme hunger (not just for food), with an inability to be satiated, correlates with Stomach and Intestinal Heat syndromes.

While, of course, we will be treating their pattern of imbalance by tonifying deficiencies, resolving excesses, and restoring the Heart-Kidney axis, an acupuncturist's role in helping wean patients off narcotics can include the National Acupuncture Detoxification Association (NADA) protocol, needling Shenmen, Lung 2, Liver, Autonomic, and Kidney points to help control cravings. These points will rarely be effective unless the patients have a strong desire to cease using the substance they are addicted to. Some recovery programs insist that a power greater than the addict must be engaged before full recovery takes place. In the meantime, our treatment principles include nourishing the Kidneys and tonifying Liver Blood, fortifying the Spleen, resolving Dampness and/or Phlegm, clearing Heat, rooting the Ming Men Fire, opening the chest, clearing the orifices, and calming the Heart-Mind. Herbal formulations such as Tian Wang Bu Xin Dang, Huang Lian E Jiao Tang, Suan Zao Ren Tang, Zhu Sha An Shen Wan, Ban Xia Huo Po Tang, and Chai Hu Jia Long Gu Mu Li Tang can help address the prominent patterns and calm the Shen while the patient faces any underlying causative factors behind the addictive behavior.

CHAPTER 6

Hypertension and Antihypertensives

Know your limits;
Don't push beyond by trying
Or you'll exhaust your Jing.

—Zhu Dan Xi

The *Tao te Ching* invites us into the depths, to be like water, and to keep our backs to the Yin, while the hurried demands of modern life have us living on the surface, burning like fire, and putting our backs up. Zhu Dan Xi, founder of the School of Nourishing Yin, stressed that our overactive Yang natures tend to burn out our Yin. This Yin isn't a substance, per se, that just dries out and is gone; it's more like the ability to be nourished from the watery depths, to unite with our source so we may be filled up with the same substance that gave us life, but isn't available to us because of our hurried lifestyles. Zhu Dan Xi believed that chronic diseases stem from over-indulgence and constrained emotions which depress the Qi and deplete the Yin so we can no longer flow like Water. He provided emotional support to his burned-out patients, relaxing the Liver with gentle herbs like Xiang Fu so the Yin organs could accept tonification. Without this approach, attempts to tonify Yin can be like flooding parched earth that just hardens in response.

Zhu Dan Xi's primary doctrine noted that Yang and Qi, which are like the sun, are often in excess; while Blood and Yin, likened to the moon, are often deficient. His second doctrine was his theory of Ministerial Fire: the Yang that is rooted in Kidney Yin is prone to being easily agitated into reckless upward movement, causing a host of emotional stirrings that move the organism out of balance. This describes the modern state of affairs—our entire planet is in a state of stirred Yang and Yin depletion. Many of our modern diseases like hypertension are due to depression, repressed emotions, over-indulgence, and burnout, manifesting in excess Yang and arterial stiffening. However, we are told, when the Ministerial Fire is informed and charged by the Sovereign Fire of the Heart, things return to balance.

> The human heart...
> put under the orders of the heart of the Tao
> is capable of being governed by stillness.

> —*Zhu Dan Xi*

One of the highest callings in Taoism is to live according to Wu Wei 無為, usually translated as non-action, which is thereby perceived as exhibiting the unappealing qualities of passivity and inertia. Yet when we let things take their own course without the interference of our willful desires, all things, including us, flow effortlessly with the natural and spontaneous movement of life. If we can cultivate a Heart-Mind in alignment with things as they are, we have access to a potency that comes from beyond the personal will.

We come into the world with all of the potential of pure Jing, and leave it exhausted of Jing, now pure Shen. And in between, Qi is the medium of exchange whereby spirit is redeemed from matter. In a world characterized by achievement and gain, we are groomed from infancy to strive for external goals. Here ambition misappropriates the gentle but powerful arising of the Zhi, the spirit of Water, and prematurely forces it into manifestation. Because this goes against nature, which does not toil to meet specific aims, our bodies have to compensate for this distorted upward and outward movement by becoming more dense, and our inner world remains hidden from view. This creates tension in the musculature, including the smooth muscles of vascular walls. Blood pressure is meant to go up and down in response to transient postural changes, external threats, and distressful emotional responses.

Cultivation practices encourage us to shift our attention from external fascination and "reverse the flow" to foster an inner awareness of how we are utilizing our Jing, Qi, and Blood. When we are rooted within our source, clear Yang ascends, and turbid Yin descends. Keeping our backs to the Yin doesn't mean turning our backs on the Yin. We can develop the capacity to look within, face, and rise above the myriad ways we may have emotionally repressed our deepest shadows. Yet balance is called for, as constant internal gazing can congeal the Yin and Blood. So we stand at the turning point where we know the Yang but abide in the Yin, and receive the world in our arms, becoming ever more fluid and lighter as we age. Alternatively, if we exhaust our Jing in pursuit of extraneous goals, we can end up unconsciously dragging around our densest energies of fear, worry, and guilt. As we continue to try to cover them over with various distractions, we may deplete and stagnate our most treasured resources. And Zhu Dan Xi noted that as Yang is stirred into reckless movement, the Qi becomes depressed, trapping Dampness, Phlegm, and Blood within. These excesses can then steam upward and cloud the orifices. This sounds like the makings of a hypertensive stroke to me.

Hypertension

The greatest danger to a man with high blood pressure lies in its discovery, because then some fool is certain to try and reduce it.

—J.H. Hay, *British Medical Journal*, 1931

In 1940, a blood pressure reading of 200 mmHg/100 mm Hg was considered mild benign hypertension, and conservative treatment was recommended, such as reassurance and weight reduction. Ten years later, the diagnostic parameters were dropped to the acceptable high range of 180/110 and doctors began to experiment with sodium restriction and dietary modifications. In the 1960s, links were made between hypertension and strokes, congestive heart failure, and kidney damage, and focus was mainly on treating diastolic blood pressure readings > 105 mmHg. In the late 1970s, large clinical trials of phar- macological research changed the landscape and about 30 antihypertensive drugs were made available. Three decades later 140/90 mmHg was considered stage 1 hypertension, and over 100 medications were marketable. Today a mean systolic blood pressure > 130 mmHg and mean diastolic blood pressure > 80 mmHg is considered hypertensive, and thus nearly half of the adult population is seen as hypertensive, the incidence increasing with age and weight. Thank heaven we have so many drugs available! Isn't it remarkable that the readings correlate with the industry's ability to meet this "need"?

Hypertension isn't a disease in itself, but a diagnosis of the pressure of affluence, sedentary lifestyles, lack of exercise, poor diet, caffeine and alcohol consumption, emotional repression, and the resultant stress on our blood vessels. Perhaps there are fewer cerebrovascular accidents now due to anti-hypertensives, but in 2022 one in six deaths from cardiovascular disease was still due to strokes, 87 percent of which were ischemic, when blood flow to the brain was blocked, not hemorrhagic strokes, where the main risk is hypertension. The global antihypertensive drug market presently yields approximately 25 billion dollars annually.

One of the body's prime directives is to ascend the Qi to ensure oxygenated blood is delivered to the brain. Kidney Yang supports Spleen Qi in its ascending function; and Kidney Yin is the source of Liver Blood, which engenders Heart Qi. Heart Qi controls the force of contraction through the Mai, whose job is to provide Blood flow to all the organ systems, extremities, and especially the Sea of Marrow. Systole governs the output of Heart Qi via Tai Yang. As the ventricles constrict, they pump blood out against the vessels, whose pressure, measured in mmHg, becomes the systolic measurement. The tremendous flow of aortic output is governed by Yang Ming. Tai Yin governs the diastolic phase, where the heart relaxes and the right ventricle refills as the pressure in the vessels falls.

The etiology of hypertension often begins with underlying pre- or postnatal tendencies toward Kidney Yin or Liver Blood deficiency. This may be constitutional; it may stem from feelings of poor self-esteem or not knowing who we are; or from an excessive lifestyle where we act beyond the capacity of our innate reserves. When the Liver Yin is exhausted and runs dry, retreat is impossible because there is nothing left within to retreat to. The Liver, which governs upbearing, coursing, and discharging, is said to be the unyielding viscus. As unfulfilled desires, frustration, resentment, anger, or any other repressed emotion damage the Liver, it loses its ability to course and discharge; the Qi stagnates and Yang becomes hyperactive, wreaking havoc on the vasculature. Add the typical American diet and lack of exercise, as well as worry and anxiety, and the Spleen and Stomach become weakened, leading to Dampness and Phlegm and obstructing the free flow of Qi, Blood, and body fluids. These Yin depressions cause Heat to swelter. Then as we age, the Kidneys become depleted; Yin fails to nourish Liver Blood, causing more Liver Qi stagnation and Heat, which consumes more Yin. As ascendant Liver Yang rises, symptoms like headaches, dizziness, bloodshot eyes, visual changes, and tinnitus are produced.

The three systems involved in maintaining pressure within the vasculature that give rise to the pathogenesis of hypertension involve the renal system, the central nervous system, and the cardiovascular systems. Any physiologic network of communication automatically involves the San Jiao mechanism as well.

- Renal involvement: In response to decreased plasma volume, blood pressure falls and sodium is reduced, stimulating renin in the kidney to convert angiotensinogen, which comes from the liver, to angiotensin 1 (AGTI). Angiotensin converting enzyme (ACE) is produced by the lungs to convert AGTI to angiotensin 2 (AGTII), which constricts arterioles and triggers the release of aldosterone from the adrenal gland, a Kidney Yang function, to cause vascular constriction and raise Liver Yang. Sodium is then reabsorbed in the kidney, increasing water retention, and circulating volume and diastolic blood pressure to increase blood pressure.

- The central nervous system: In order to maintain constant pressure for blood to circulate, changes in posture activate baroreceptors in the walls of the aorta and carotid artery that cause transitory shifts in the Qi mechanism. This increases the sympathetic nervous system's constriction of blood vessels, deactivates the peripheral nervous system which causes vasodilation, and triggers the release of norepinephrine (Kidney Yang). This contracts the vasculature, raising Liver Yang, Heart Qi, and systolic output, in order to increase peripheral blood flow.

- Cardiac involvement: Each time the heart contracts, the force of Yang Ming pounds against the inside of the ventricular and arteriolar walls. As the heart pumps against this pressure, the cardiac muscle can hypertrophy, causing thickening in the ventricular walls, and heart enlargement, while the pressure builds up in the vasculature.

These three mechanisms result from deeper imbalances beneath the surface. We all repress the myriad ways our systems are bombarded by overwhelm, whether it be from childhood trauma or day-to-day stressors. One of the most helpful tools at our disposal is to support our patients in becoming aware of how their lifestyle impacts their physiology. Slowing down allows us to remain present to the signs our bodies convey. Psychological studies have reported that emotional defensiveness, under which lie unexpressed emotions that we are unaware of, is linked to hypertension. This is particularly true of the population that seems upbeat all the time, regardless of what problems they encounter. The conscious mind doesn't erase the effects of trauma, and the body reveals what unexpressed emotions can't. While our constitutional makeup gives rise to these repressive tendencies, excess weight exacerbates their expression.

The way we move our bodies is important. When we are instructed to exercise, we may resist images of sweating at the gym, lifting weights, running around a track, or getting on an exercise bike. But healthy body movement can be so much more than that. All that's required is it is enjoyable, invigorating, and helps us to experience more flow in our bodies. Instead of going to the gym, some people might prefer dancing, playing outside, hiking, or doing somersaults down a hill. Qi Gong, grounding, and earthing practices are also helpful ways to engage the body's ability to subdue excess Yang and calm internal Wind. Clearing excess fats, refined carbohydrates, sugar, and dairy from the diet can also help. Additionally, foods like beets have high nitrate levels, which the body converts into nitric oxide, a vasodilator that relaxes the vasculature and lowers blood pressure. But if we are to address the root, the patient's consciousness must be part of the treatment. Help them to remain present with their own inner experience. While we may be the ones treating blood pressure elevations, they are the ones who resolve them.

Common patterns that may result in elevated blood pressure often include an underlying Liver Blood and Kidney Yin deficiency, which gives rise to ascendant Liver Yang or Liver Fire. Further, Spleen Qi vacuity may result in Dampness and Phlegm, and long-standing Qi stagnation leads to Blood stasis. In addition to treating the particular pattern, acupuncture points which reduce blood pressure include Ki 1, Lv 2, Lv 3, Ll 4, St 9, Ht 7, GB 39, GB 43, and Ren 5, and bleeding Erjian at the ear apex. While patterns may be more complex, our treatment principles to lower pressure may include the following:

- Harmonizing the Liver and subduing Yang (Long Dan Xie Can Tang, Tian Ma Gou Teng Yin): GB 38, Lv 3, Ki 3, GB 20, St 36, Ll 11.
- Clearing Gallbladder Damp Heat or Phlegm Fire disturbing the Heart (Huang Lian Wen Dan Tang): Lv 3, GB 20, St 36, Ll 11, GB 44.
- Calming internal Wind (Tian Ma Gou Teng Yin): GB 20, Du 16, Lv 8.
- Sedating and calming the spirit (Chai Hu Jia Long Gu Mu Li Tang): Pc 6, Pc 8.
- Harmonizing the Liver and Spleen (Chai Hu Shu Gan Tang): Sp 6, St 36, Lv 3, Lv 13.
- Harmonizing Shao Yang (Da Chai Hu Tang): GB 39, SJ 5.
- Tonifying underlying Kidney Yin and Liver Blood vacuity, and clear deficient Heat (Liu Wei di Huang Wan, Zhi Bai di Huang Wan): Ki 3, Sp 6, Lv 8, GB 39, St 36.

Phlegm may be a complicating factor in chronic hypertensive scenarios and Ban Xia Bai Zhu Tian Ma Tang might be appropriate. Blood stasis can also complicate hypertension, and blood thinners are often prescribed, which deplete Kidney Yang. We can tonify Kidney Yang to move the Blood or add Blood-invigorating medicinals such as Xue Fu Zhu Yu Tang, Tao Ren, and Hong Hua. UB 17 can also redirect reckless blood flow through the aorta and vena cava by regulating the diaphragm.

The *Shen Nong Ben Cao* tells us that the upper class of medicines govern the nourishment of destiny and correspond to Heaven. Thus, if one wishes to prolong the years of life without aging, one should use these. The middle class of medicines govern the nourishment of one's nature and correspond to humanity. If, then, one wishes to prevent illness and to supplement depletions and emaciations, one should use these. The lower class of medicines govern the treatment of illness and correspond to Earth. If one wishes to remove Cold, Heat, and other evil influences from the body, to break accumulations, and to cure illnesses, one should base one's efforts on drugs listed in the lower class.

If we were nourishing our destiny with the upper class of medicines, we would probably not be interested in reading about antihypertensives. We might, however, ingest substances that foster grounding and meditation, as we detach from materiality and humbly enter the dark inner caves until the luminous darkness of Yin begins to glow. If we were nourishing our nature to prevent the development of illnesses, we would be addressing the patterns listed above before hypertension arose. And if we were attempting to cure the hypertensive illness, we might utilize herbs that are known to regulate blood pressure, such as Shan Zha, Ge Gen, Xia Ku Cao, Ye Ju Hua, Long Kui, Long Dan Cao, Han Fang Ji, Yu Mi Xu, Xi Xian Cao, Ma Dou Ling, Sang Ji Sheng, Du Zhong, Yin Yang Huo, Yi Mu Cao, Da Ji, Shan Zhu Yu, Gou Teng, Shi Jue Ming, and Shan Zha.

Herbs which have a diuretic effect include Bai Zhu, Che Qian Cao, Che Qian Zi, Cang Zhu, Da Huang, Dan Zhu Ye, Dang Gui, Du Zhong, Fu Ling, Gui Zhi, Huang Qi, Huang Qin, Jie Geng, Jin Qian Cao, Ku Shen, Lian Qiao, Ma Huang, Mao Gen, Mu Tong, Qin Pi, Qu Mai, San Qi, Sang Ji Sheng, Shu Di, Yin Chen, Yu Mi Xu, Yu Xing Cao, Ze Xie, Zhi Qiao, and Zhu Ling.

Antihypertensive drugs

Drugs to lower blood pressure fall into three main categories that target the three main causative mechanisms:

- Diuretics, which act primarily on the kidneys.
- Anti-adrenergics that impact the nervous system's control of the heart.
- Vasodilators, which act on the blood vessels to reduce vascular pressure.

Diuretics

Diuretics cause the kidneys to increase renal output via various mechanisms. Similar to herbs which drain Dampness like Fu Ling and Zhu Ling, they are meant to reduce circulating blood volume. Depending on the specific diuretic prescribed, this category of pharmaceuticals can disrupt fluid metabolism and injure the Yin, decrease glucose tolerance, and raise cholesterol—signs that Dampness is compensating for Yin vacuity. The pulses may be fine and weak, or slippery.

THIAZIDE DIURETICS

- Chlorothiazide (Diuril)
- Metolazone (Zaroxolyn)
- Hydrochlorothiazide (Microzide, Esidrix Aquazide h)
- Chlorthalidone (Thalitone)
- Metolazone (Mykrox)
- Indapamide (Lozol)
- Methylclothiazide (Enduron, Aquatensen)

Thiazide diuretics inhibit the reabsorption of sodium and chloride ions in the kidneys' distal tubules. Urine output increases, and the loss of sodium reduces the glomerular filtration rate. Potassium and chloride are dumped along with it. These diuretics also cause vasodilation, which reduces pressure on the heart and vessels. Side effects are largely due to the electrolyte imbalances. As Na+, K+, and Cl– are reduced, hypercalcemia, hyperglycemia, hyperlipidemia, hyperuricemia, and metabolic alkalosis may result. These include weakness, back, leg, or stomach pains, GI distress, bloating, black tarry or clay-colored stools, chest pain, dizziness, hypotension, blue lips and fingernails, sun sensitivity, reduced urine output, gout, and renal insufficiency. Thiazides are often used in patients with normal Kidney function, although they do carry a high risk. The draining action of these diuretics can deplete the Yin and disrupt fluid metabolism, reducing and stagnating the Qi and fluids. This can result in Dampness, and Cold, stasis, and organ failure.

LOOP DIURETICS

- Furosemide (Lasix)
- Ethacrynic acid (Ethacrynate, Edecrin)

- Torsemide (Demadex, Soaanz)
- Bumetanide (Bumex)

Loop diuretics also inhibit electrolyte absorption in the kidneys, but in the ascending loop of Henle. More often prescribed for patients with impaired renal function, they are more potent than the thiazides. Thus, the results of fluid depletion and electrolyte imbalances are magnified. Similar to the side effects listed above, low blood volume, headaches, dizziness, and ototoxicity, including tinnitus and deafness, may result.

POTASSIUM-SPARING DIURETICS

- Amiloride (Midamor)
- Spironolactone (Aldactone, CaroSpir)
- Eplerenone (Inspra)
- Triamterene (Dyrenium)

Potassium-sparing diuretics, like their name suggests, increases the excretion of sodium while holding onto potassium. Potassium drives energy out of the cell, while sodium drives energy into the cell. Sodium causes an upward movement; potassium causes more expansion. Thus, as sodium is reduced but potassium is not, we see a reduction in the ascending action of sodium. In addition to lowering blood pressure, these diuretics are also prescribed to treat edema, congestive heart failure, hyperaldosteronism, cirrhosis, and nephrotic syndrome. Potential side effects include reduced urination and hypovolemia. The increased potassium levels (hyperkalemia) can cause an increase in circulating water in the chest, resulting in slowing of the heart, respiratory distress, chest pain, and renal dysfunction. Symptoms also include increased thirst, confusion, vomiting, and increased urination.

OSMOTIC DIURETICS
Mannitol (Resectisol): Osmotic diuretics inhibit the reabsorption of sodium and water, to draw water into the urine. Used to reduce intracranial pressure and swelling in the eye, mannitol initially increases plasma volume and blood pressure, drawing intracellular water out of the brain and into the blood

and finally out through the urine. This has a mildly dehydrating effect on the brain. It is also prescribed for those with acute renal failure to remove toxins from the body. Side effects include headache, nausea, vomiting, chills, dizziness, lethargy, confusion, chest pain, and polydipsia.

All of these diuretics reduce fluid volume and excess pressure by draining fluid downward in varying degrees. Hypertensive states are rarely caused by excess fluid however, but by Liver depression stagnating the Qi and causing Yang to rise. Thus, you can see that diuretics can reduce blood pressure without addressing the source. The resulting drainage can disrupt fluid metabolism, causing dryness, damaging Yin, and upsetting the dynamics between Spleen and Stomach Qi. Our treatments will need to tonify Yin, Blood, and Qi as appropriate, restore fluids, harmonize Qi, and address the underlying pattern of imbalance that gave rise to the hypertensive state.

Antiadrenergics

The term adrenergic denotes the effects of the adrenal neurotransmitters epinephrine and norepinephrine. These chemicals cause Yang Qi to rise by activating the sympathetic nervous system, constricting blood vessels and stimulating the heart to beat faster. These effects represent how Kidney Yang supports the Spleen Qi in ascending, as well as how Kidney and Liver Yin finance Liver Blood, which engenders Heart Qi. The mechanisms involve the Heart-Kidney axis and the San Jiao. Some antiadrenergics act on the central nervous system's alpha-adrenergic receptors, which cause smooth muscles in the vasculature to contract, resulting in blood pressure elevations. Beta-adrenergic receptors relax smooth muscles and cause vasodilation, but also have an excitatory effect on the heart. The antiadrenergic class of drugs inhibit the release of adrenergic agonists, or antagonize their receptors. The alpha- and betablocking effects then reduce blood pressure and cardiac output by blocking the Kidney output, reducing Liver Yang rising and Heart Qi.

CENTRAL ACTING ANTIADRENERGICS

- Guanfacine (Intuniv, Tenex)
- Clonidine (Catapres, Kapvay, Nexiclon XR, Duraclon)
- Lofexidine (Lucemyra)

- Methyldopa (Aldomet)
- Guanabenz (Wytensin)

These drugs block the release and action of epinephrine, norepinephrine, and dopamine, and inhibit stimulation of the alpha-adrenergic receptors, which results in a decrease in vasoconstriction and cardiac output. Reducing Yang output and impairing Liver Blood's ability to engender Heart Qi induces the side effects, which include drowsiness, sedation, headaches, impotence, and impaired ejaculation. Blocking the Liver can disturb the Hun, resulting in involuntary movements, nightmares, and psychic disturbance—common signs when dopamine regulation is altered. The San Jiao's Fire-Water action can be impeded, disrupting fluid metabolism and distribution and causing dry mouth, while the rashes and involuntary movements can be caused by the resulting Heat and Wind.

BETABLOCKERS

- Acebutolol (Sectral)
- Atenolol (Tenormin)
- Bisoprolol (Monocor)
- Carvedilol (Coreg)
- Labetalol (Trandate)
- Metoprolol (Lopressor, Betaloc)
- Nadolol (Corgard)
- Pindolol (Viskazide)
- Propranolol (Inderal)
- Timolol (Blocadren)

Beta-adrenergic blocking agents inhibit the effects of epinephrine and nor-epinephrine at the cellular receptor sites. This reduces the beta sympathetic nervous system response, decreasing cardiac contractions. In addition to lowering blood pressure, they reduce abnormal heart rhythms and treat angina. Because they also cause narrowing of the airways, bronchospasm is one of the side effects. Others include bradycardia, fatigue, bad dreams, and hallucinations. They can also lower Co-enzyme Q10 and magnesium levels, and the imbalance can cause bowel and sleep disturbances. Their mechanism of action involves blocking Kidney Yang, which reduces Heart Qi and Yang. Heart Yang, being unable to transport Blood to the extremities, can result in cold hands and feet. The Qi may also stagnate in the chest. The pulse will often be weak, deep, and slow, manifesting the resultant Yang deficiency.

We can restore Heart-Kidney communication, restore Qi flow in the chest, invigorate the Yang with moxibustion to help reduce some of the side effects, and harmonize the Liver.

Vasodilators

Vasoconstriction is a Yang Qi effect induced by stimulatory neurotransmitters like norepinephrine, stress, and stimulants like caffeine. Vasodilators counter the Yang action of vasoconstriction and thereby relax the blood vessels.

ACE INHIBITORS

- Benazepril (Lotensin)
- Captopril (Capoten)
- Enalapril/enalaprilat (Vasotec oral and injectable)
- Fosinopril (Monopril)
- Lisinopril (Zestril and Prinivil)
- Moexipril (Univasc)
- Oerindopril (Aceon)
- Quinapril (Accupril)
- Ramipril (Altace)
- Trandolapril (Mavik)

Reviewing the renal mechanism of hypertension, when plasma volume decreases, blood pressure and sodium levels fall. Because we still need to get blood to the brain, renin from the kidneys is stimulated to convert angiotensinogen from the Liver into AGT1. Angiotensin-converting enzyme (ACE) converts the less active AGT1 to the active AGTII, causing Kidney Yang to constrict arterioles and trigger the release of aldosterone from the adrenal gland. Sodium is reabsorbed in the kidneys, causing an increase in water retention, circulating volume, and diastolic blood pressure. We can view this process as Kidney Yang giving rise to Liver Yang rising.

ACE inhibitors block the conversion of AGTI to AGTII, thereby preventing the vasoconstrictive effects of AGTII. The enzyme inhibition increases potassium levels going to the blood vessels, which relaxes the vessels. Hypotension results, as well as decreased renal perfusion. This blocking effect can lead to deteriorating renal function, and mineral imbalances which affect the Kidneys. This Kidney suppression doesn't allow the ascending action of Qi, resulting in deficient-type side effects such as fatigue, headache, and dizziness from lowered perfusion to the head. The resulting hypotension can also cause rebound tachycardia. ACE is produced in the pulmonary endothelium, and ACE inhibitors can produce a mild dry cough and lost of taste, as their effects impair the Lung-Kidney interaction. The pulse will often be fine and weak.

CALCIUM CHANNEL BLOCKERS

- Amlodipine (Norvasc, Norliqva, Katerzia)
- Clevidipine (Cleviprex)
- Diltiazem (Cartia XT, Cardizem, Cardizem CD, Cardizem LA, Tiazac, Taztia XT, Dilacor XR, Tiadylt ER, Matzim LA, Diltzac, Diltia XT)
- Felodipine (Plendil)
- Isradipine (Dynacirc CR, Dynacirc)
- Levamlodipine (Conjupri)
- Nicardipine (Cardene, Cardene SR, Cardene IV)
- Nifedipine (Adalat, Adalat CC, Procardia, Procardia XL, Nifedical XL, Nifediac CC, Afeditab CR)
- Nimodipine (Nimotop, Nymalize)
- Nisoldipine (Sular)
- Verapamil (Calan, Calan SR, Verelan, Covera-HS)

Calcium is our main alkalinizing agent and plays a role in bone metabolism (Kidney function), protein absorption (Stomach), muscular contraction (Spleen), transmission of nerve impulses (San Jiao), fat transfer (Spleen/ Liver), blood clotting (Spleen/Liver), and cardiac function (Heart). Calcium ion channels cause muscular contractions within the heart and blood vessels.

Calcium channel blockers prevent the influx of calcium into the muscle cells of blood vessel walls. Disrupting the movement of calcium through the channels causes arteriolar dilation and reduced blood pressure. This also prevents the contraction of the cardiac muscle, slowing the heart rate, allowing the left ventricle to fill completely between systolic contractions, thereby reducing the heart's workload. The left side of the heart distributes Heart Qi, a Tai Yang function.

Calcium channel blockers also inhibit smooth muscle propulsion in the GI tract, which can cause constipation. Other side effects include nausea, stomach upset, weakness, fatigue, light headedness, dizziness, headaches, sweating, palpitations, hypotension, bradycardia, flushing, edema, cough, stuffy nose, and sore throat. Because of the reduced contraction of the vasculature and increased arteriolar dilation, the tension required for proper Qi interaction is diminished. This decrease in Qi can injure both the Kidney Yang and Heart Blood. As Yang Qi is subdued, movement of Heart Qi is slowed. The increase in vasodilation vents Blood and Heat to the surface, resulting in local flushing to the skin and respiratory mucosa.

When one is taking antihypertensives to reduce blood pressure because of heart conditions, stimulants like caffeine should be avoided. Ma Huang is contraindicated with antihypertensives, because its stimulating effect dilates the chest and lifts up the Wei Qi. Kidney Yang deficiency might be the pattern behind hypertension, and stimulants weaken Kidney Yang, thus worsening hypertension. Mild Kidney astringent herbs like Wu Wei Zi can be helpful.

A 46-year-old politician had been diagnosed with hypertension in college. His only other relevant medical history included low back pain and low sperm count. He had been on Losartin Potassium (Cozaar), an angiotensin II receptor antagonist which controlled his hypertension, but made him dizzy and short of breath. The medication, which relaxes the blood vessels, made it difficult to breathe, he coughed a lot, and experienced some tingling in his feet. He did not want to remain on the prescription, but his doctors had never given him another option. He thought he would have to remain on some sort of antihypertensive medication for the rest of his life. I told him I would treat his pattern and we could see how his blood pressure responded. While I expected to see ascendant Liver Yang as his presenting pattern, it was not. His diagnosis included Kidney Yang and Spleen Qi deficiency, with floating Yang, and only mild Liver Qi stagnation. His Kidneys needed tonification so they could root the Yang. I needled GB 21, Lv 3, LI 4, and Ren 4 with moxa. He was prescribed a formula with Dang Shen, Yin Yang Huo, Du Zhong, Chai Hu Da Zao, Zhi Shi, Bai Shao, Mu Li, and Rou Gui. His blood pressure lowered almost immediately, and he was advised to decrease his medication. Within a month, he was able to wean off the Cozaar altogether.

CHAPTER 7

Anti-Diabetic Drugs

Be the Valley
So the whole Universe
Comes to you

Dynamics of digestion

Receptivity is a state of emptiness represented by the "Valley Spirit," situated so lowly that no effort is required as Heaven pours its life-giving powers into it. The *Book of Rites* says:

> The Qi of earth ascends, the Qi of heaven descends. In this fashion, Yin and Yang grind against each other, and Heaven and Earth merge in undulating embrace. If this setting is vibrated by thunder, excited by wind and rain, moved by the flow of the four seasons, and fondled by the germinating light of sun and moon, the world's myriad processes of transformation become aroused.

Everything comes from emptiness. The *Nei Jing* describes Yin and Yang as the root and origin of life and death, yet they form *but a playing field for the mysterious process of visible manifestation emerging from an invisible center.*

The Celestial Qi descends, to be received by the invisible center in the hollow Fu organs that transmit from above to below. Therefore, the Way of Heaven is to empty ourselves like the bowels. In suit, the six Fu transform, drain, and empty, but do not store. All physical phenomena emerge from the empty center, but have to be banked into existence. Storage belongs to the Zang organs, which come from Earth and reach upward. For some reason, perhaps because we want to perpetuate our finite forms, humans prefer storing things up rather than the process of emptying them out. And in the modern Western world, the majority of chronic disease states are associated with overly storing, and not enough transformation, draining, and emptying.

The value of emptying and filling was established in-utero. The cosmic embrace of our Earthly mother and Heavenly father conceived us in our divine perfection. Ren Mai carries the Heart of the Mother, which Du Mai vitalizes with Yang Qi. During the second trimester of gestation, when Shen were imparting our curriculum, it is said that Heaven blew six unique pitches of vibration through each of the newly developing and still empty Fu organs—a mysterious melody of the soul, reminding us of our origin and our destiny before we were birthed into being. Always there, hidden deeply in the invisible center in the bowels, our distinct celestial song remains to be discovered. *There's a hidden sweetness in the stomach's emptiness*, said Rumi. *We are lutes, to be burned clean with fasting...* until a new song arises. It seems as if we were born with a deep aspiration, longing, and hope for something eternal. Yet when our desires become displaced only for things of the Earth, we end up becoming saturated with more food, drink, and thinking than we need. As we hunger for more to fill up the emptiness, we become deafened to the cosmic notes that beckon us home, and often need to empty ourselves of excess clutter before we can recognize these subtle vibrations.

Our ability to take in the world in its various forms belongs to the concept of receptivity, the primal Yin principle that belongs to the intrinsic Yin channel, Ren Mai. The conception vessel establishes our necessary earthly survival functions like eating, drinking, bonding, and the ability to be nourished by life to sustain life. Ren Mai gives us our sense of belonging to ourselves, to fully receive this earthly life, to need others, and to be needed. Kidney Yin functions according to the dictates set forth by the Conception energetics— our ability to take in, to be satiated, and the sense of inner certainty that comes from how we receive ourselves. Ren Mai governs the development and coordination of the circular muscles around the eyes and mouth, the sphincters of the throat, esophagus, and stomach, and the intestinal movements throughout the gut tube—initiating primal peristaltic wave-like rhythms, propelled downward by gravity and Wei Qi. Arranged in horizontal segments as vertical conduits of energy for intake, expression, exchange, and release, these primitive circular mechanisms may become locked up through control, repression, suppression, and armoring. More primal than the nervous system, they are part of the ancestral sinews, which give rise to the parasympathetic process of digestion. Ren Mai initiates the descending movement of Gu Qi via the suckling instinct. As the teeth emerge, the more complex functional dynamic of breaking down food particles will be taken over by the Stomach official, who will decompose and downbear the turbid contents of digestion so the five Zang can receive their boons.

Chong Mai is the next evolutionary channel involved with digestion and metabolism that unites the Conception and Governing Vessels to establish the blueprint on which the Mandate of Heaven, Tian Ming, will be carried out. The Penetrating Meridian provides the bridge by which our prenatal dynamics, the cards we were dealt, are conditioned into a postnatal life narrative. Chong Mai wraps together the spiraling genetic sequence of the Yin and Yang components of Jing to communicate precisely how to bank the Qi and Blood in support of its ability to raise the heaviness of Earth as we walk through life. Chong Mai is animated with a great power to correctly circulate Qi and Blood as the seed of potential of the lower burner ascends to the ancestral Qi in the chest. The first ancestry of Chong Mai, from Ki 11 to Ki 21, represents how we assimilate and digest life in order to condition the Blood with Shen. It gives rise to both the Kidneys and the Stomach, evidenced by St 30, Qi Chong, as its meeting point.

As the Stomach meridian runs from the eye to the mouth and around the jaw before plunging into the gut, it constitutes the rudimentary reception between our environment and our sensory apparatus. It is the pathway through which information enters the body-mind, before we assign specific meaning to it. The Stomach is basic for survival; the whole of our flesh wraps around this out-pouching of the gut tube, which breaks things down for initial processing, out of which our physical body, especially the musculature, will be fashioned, since the Stomach is in charge of digesting protein. The Stomach's rotting and ripening process conveys the idea of breaking things down so they can become something else. The way we absorb information and synthesize experiences prior to personally ascribing any emotional significance is the Stomach's psychological equivalent.

The Spleen, on the other hand, will provide meaning to that which the Stomach has taken in. In the same way that Gu Qi becomes Blood, our experiences, when fully assimilated, become our life narrative, a summary of ideas on which our beliefs and views of life are based. Too much or the wrong type of food, information, or stress simply can't be absorbed. When input exceeds the Stomach's capacity to process, digestive disorders, abdominal fullness, and cluttered thoughts are likely to ensue. We could say the Stomach receives each event purely without context—it simply breaks things down for initial digestion. Then the more complex and earthy Spleen steps in to define what it means for the individual, interpreting based on past associations and beliefs. If the Spleen is bogged down with overthinking, the Qi mechanism may become knotted up, the gut and neurotransmitters become clogged with Dampness, our receptors may malfunction, and, as the messages aren't being conveyed clearly, we are left confused and foggy headed. We might be filled up, but to no avail.

Further, fluid metabolism begins with the Stomach, the origin of fluids, which sends clear liquids to the sensory orifices and to the Spleen for distribution to the rest of the body. The turbid fluids pass to the Small Intestine, which plunges into the depths and again separates the thin pure fluids from the impure, allowing what, according to the discernment given by the Heart, will enter into the Blood.

When the Stomach and Spleen are not able to keep up with their physical or psychological duties, our metabolic performance may malfunction. Here we have to look at how much we are consuming and why, and whether or not we are taking in more than we can metabolize and utilize. The Stomach governs hunger, and establishes the foundation of how the Spleen will process and distribute the Gu Qi into usable energy. Hunger and thirst for food and drink, cravings for physical and non-physical satiation, and longings for emotional or spiritual fulfillment form a spectrum which crosses from the Spleen/Stomach to the Liver/Gallbladder. The primary disharmony of the Gallbladder is Damp Heat accumulation, which arises from the Spleen's failure to transform and transport; that is, to process the fulfillment of our desires into usable Qi, which can then obstruct the Liver and Gallbladder.

Faulty sugar metabolism and the development of metabolic syndrome, glucose intolerance, insulin resistance, and diabetes

Exocrine glands excrete their substances to external surfaces like the skin and gut; endocrine glands secrete hormones directly into the bloodstream. The pancreas functions as both. It is an exocrine gland as it secretes enzymes into the small intestine to digest protein, fat, and sugar. It is also an endocrine gland because its beta cells release insulin and glucagon into the bloodstream to regulate blood sugar. These processes describe transformation and transportation, the Yang Qi functions of the Spleen.

Humans have moved beyond our original hunter-gatherer diet, which sustained us for about a million years, made up of whole animals, nuts, seeds, roots, and fruits. Within the last ten to twelve thousand years, though, humans developed the capacity to expand their diets to include dairy and grains. Fast forward to this last century when we started consuming concentrated sugars, preservatives, breads, and animal fat, while developing sedentary lifestyles that lead to overthinking and hungering for more than we need. This has wreaked havoc on our internal organs, especially the dynamics of the Spleen. Our propensity for sweets was initially a mechanism to fuel survival as this quick energy source keeps us hypervigilant to stressors which may threaten us. Since we no longer require rapid bursts of sugar in order to survive, most of us now equate sweetness with kindness and comfort, of being loved, nurtured, and cared for. But this level of nourishment is a function that belongs to the Conception meridian, and should ultimately be self-sourced. If we are unable to meet this internal need ourselves, we tend to project it onto others, and may be seen as sickly or needy. They may need to distance themselves, making the individual become either more Yin deficient or prone to Yin stasis and Phlegmy conditions. Further, compensatory attempts to provide for those around us at our own expense weakens the Spleen and creates Dampness, causing pathological conditions to linger. Refined and immediately available sugar temporarily and superficially gives us a feeling of satisfaction, perhaps temporarily satiating a deeper need to belong to a larger place in the nature of the cosmic order. Maybe this is why we are so addicted to sweetness; yet it leaves a filmy residue in its wake, reminding us that Earth alone will never satisfy our need for knowing Heaven within. Yes, what we eat matters. But why we eat what we eat often matters more.

We eat to provide fuel for the body, but our receptors also hunger for intangible things. Like the function of SI 19, *Palace of Inner Listening*, if you listen deep enough into the Heart-Mind to access the emptiness, there is a longing for something subtly and intangibly pure that no amount of food, drink, or neurotransmitter adjusting can fulfill.

The Spleen/pancreas represents our affinity for sweetness, and the ability to transform Gu Qi into enfleshed energy. When glucose enters the blood-stream, the pancreas releases insulin, the storage hormone responsible for Spleen's transformation (Qi) and transportation (Yang) functions. Earth banks the glucose by utilizing insulin (Spleen Yang) to drive sugar into the cell to be utilized. The pancreas (whose Shu point is UB 17.5) also produces gluca-gon, which opposes the actions of insulin by stimulating the liver to release glucose that has been stored as glycogen in order to raise blood sugar levels. This is one of the ways that Liver/Spleen harmony is maintained. Pancreatic function also plays a role in modulating adrenal activity. In response to short-term stressors, adrenaline, a Kidney Yang hormone, is released, which is then countered by the Dampening effects of cortisol, which attempts to prevent blood sugar spikes and falls, and this can ultimately be quite stressful to the system.

Because every cell relies on glucose, all edible food substance is seen to be at least somewhat "sweet," even if its dominant taste is salty or sour, so it can be recognized and processed by the Spleen/pancreas as fuel. Furthermore, all refined carbohydrates break down to glucose, which is the main source of cellular energy used to make ATP. The functioning of key organs critical to survival like the brain, liver, and kidneys relies on the maintenance of proper blood sugar levels.

The process of reception begins even before food enters the Stomach to become Gu Qi. The sensation of hunger may trigger the thought of food and then the sight and smell stimulate salivary enzymes to anticipate the digestive process. Even thoughts such as "I want a candy bar" may trigger the senses, and stimulate hunger for something sweet. Whether the candy is sweetened with sugar, Sucralose, fructose, or Stevia, sweet-taste receptors (GLP-1) on the tongue initiate insulin and/or glucagon release from the pancreas, and signal the gut to activate the appropriate enzymes and bacteria to digest the contents. All sweets tell the gut flora to prepare for a glucose meal. When sugar doesn't arrive, the entire system is thrown off. The activated enzymes and bacteria have nothing to act on, but remain alert, sometimes triggering more sweet cravings. This seems to be the mechanism whereby artificial sweeteners have been found to alter the intestinal microbiome and lead to glucose intolerance.

The germs in our gut influence our brain chemistry. Ongoing bidirectional communication occurs between the brain and the gut and there are more than a hundred million nerve cells via the vagus nerve, a process by which the gut microbiome is involved in influencing your thoughts, moods, and behavior. Intestinal bacteria are responsible for generating the majority of neurotransmitter functions: 90–95 percent of serotonin and about half of our dopamine stores are produced in the gut, as well as norepinephrine, GABA, and acetylcholine. When we are stressed, our inner landscape is stressed too, agitating bacteria that generate the chemicals which cause immune-modulating and inflammatory mediators, right along with their ability to produce states of depression and anxiety. If it's important to listen to our gut, it's equally important to provide our gut with adequate sustenance to maintain inner harmony.

Diets high in sugar deactivate our taste receptors while dampening the effect of dopamine, the neurotransmitter that makes us feel satiated. Dopamine plays a role in regulating blood sugar and the release of insulin, as well as helping to protect the mucosal lining of the stomach. Interestingly, one of the effects of GB 34 is to normalize the neurotransmission of dopamine; perhaps one of the mechanisms whereby in addition to treating Phlegm Heat that hinders Stomach descension, it can also address the *gnawing fear of being apprehended*, a unique behavioral reaction that likely involves an imbalance in neurotransmitters.

When glucose, the sweet Yin substance that provides the Yang energy needed by all cells, is taken in, insulin transports it into the cell or banks it for later use. When glucose is in abundance, it taxes the Spleen Yang's ability to drive it into the cell to be utilized. The excess accumulates as Dampness in the Blood, while the cells remain deprived of the sugar they need. The untransformed Gu Qi creates a Damp and sticky environment, prone to stagnation and Heat, which requires more water to flush out the excess. This diverts the Kidney energies away from their other crucial functions so they may assist in transformation, a process which drains our foundational resources and can ultimately result in Kidney deficiency, increased urination, and thirst. Epinephrine, cortisol, and thyroxine also increase blood glucose levels, giving rise to Liver-Spleen disharmony, and as the Liver Qi becomes more congested, depressive Heat may result. Sugar has an inflammatory effect, making the body more acidic, which has a corrosive effect on the delicate vascular walls. To prevent the Heat from damaging the system, it may retain Dampness. And since we still have to go on expending Yang Qi to utilize the sugar as our energy supply, this energy under pressure can produce a rather combustible environment. The stickiness of the blood causes blood cells to aggregate together, which equates with Blood stagnation, inhibiting proper circulation and functioning of the heart, kidneys, and brain. Meanwhile, the cells themselves are not able to receive their primary source of fuel, which causes them to malfunction.

Our unhealthy attempts to satiate hunger can give rise to a condition called "metabolic syndrome," a modern description of a cluster of risk factors resulting from the faulty metabolism described above. The impairment of the Spleen's transformation and transportation functions then can manifest as elevated blood sugar levels, hypertension, reduced high density lipoprotein (HDL) cholesterol, elevated low density lipoprotein (LDL) cholesterol or triglyceride levels, hypothyroid, adrenal fatigue, and increased waist circumference.

Metabolic syndrome tends to develop in Damp, sticky, and stagnant environments that correlate with many common, chronic disease processes, including heart disease, atherosclerosis, organ failure, and senility. It also provides the perfect sticky environment ripe for inhabitation by Gu and Gui. Conventional medicine and psychotherapeutic remedies simply cannot keep up with this colossal affliction of our modern lifestyle. As pharmaceuticals and their doctors chase around the effects, the root cause remains safely hidden underground.

Hyperglycemia is a condition of excess seen in pre-diabetic scenarios. The mechanism underlying the blood sugar elevations is known as glucose intolerance, where increased blood sugar causes excess storage in the form of Dampness or fat. Doctors like to see normal fasting blood glucose levels below 100 mg/dL. If consistently higher, it means the excess sugar isn't being burned off, so it lingers, plugging up hepatic receptors and causing fatty livers, and the excess in the sinews can lead to muscular weakness. This state is also associated with chronic inflammation, as the excess sugar combined with the Yang of insulin forms Heat toxins, which can then call out more cholesterol to dampen the Fire, a process which produces atherosclerosis and increases the risk of cardiovascular disease and stroke. Associated patterns include Dampness, Heat, Qi stagnation, Phlegm, and Blood stasis.

Hemoglobin A1C measurements refer to glycosylated hemoglobin, or how many sugar molecules are stuck on the blood cells. Over a red blood cell's 120-day lifespan, glucose combines with hemoglobin to produce gly-cohemoglobin, so this test provides a long-term average of the amount of glucose present in the bloodstream over a four-month period, making it more reliable than a single fasting blood glucose level. Hemoglobin A1C assesses the Spleen Qi and Yang's transformation and transportation function and its propensity for Damp accumulation. Elevated HbA1C levels indicate how well Spleen Yang is functioning, how much Dampness may accumulate, and the likelihood of further complications of Heat, Phlegm, Stagnation, and Stasis.

Fasting insulin levels provide the most accurate readings for pancreatic function, as this test measures the amount of insulin produced by pancreatic beta cells to determine the need for insulin replacement in Type I diabetic patients. Insulin levels measure the functioning of Spleen Yang, and the Liver's ability to regulate Qi. High insulin levels are associated with Dampness, Phlegm, Heat, and Qi stagnation, all of which impair the Spleen and Liver Qi's ability to transport glucose into the cells for utilization.

In Type II diabetes, cells lose the ability to recognize or respond to insulin anymore, creating a condition known as insulin resistance. As the sticky and inflammatory sugar levels rise, insulin (Spleen Yang) levels also rise to try to drive out or transport the sugar elsewhere. As insulin tries harder to get the cell walls to open up to receive the glucose, the excess Yang acts like a fiery solvent to the interior epithelial lining of blood vessel walls, eventually weakening and predisposing them to tears. The liver then sends out more LDL to blanket the fragile lining, and cholesterol becomes trapped in the repair. Spleen (and Kidney) Yang weakens, Damp Heat accumulates, and Yin becomes depleted. This is a setup for blood cholesterol elevations, which often stems from the inflammation caused by the hot, sticky environment created by glucose intolerance. Combined with hypertension, we have the perfect storm of conditions for many of our most debilitating chronic diseases.

Xiao Ke, wasting and thirsting disorder, is associated with simple sugar and carbohydrate consumption which accumulates as Dampness, creating an environment conducive to development of Heat, which dries out the Yin. The Rehmannia formulas are great for tonifying underlying Yin, Qi, and Blood deficiency and addressing Dampness. In the Western world, however, our diets tend to have higher levels of protein and therefore Heat, which then causes Damp to accumulate, giving rise to a unique type of obesity with underlying Heat sweltering. This Heat can damage the fluid and electrolyte balance, and a more recent addition, Jade Spring, is better for restoring hydration. As the accumulated sugar thickens the Blood, Damp and Phlegm can collect in the kidney tubules. They may become irritated, and their linings become constricted by the inflammation, which can then lead to back flow into the prostate or bladder, producing swelling and constriction. More water is required to dilute the sugar, so we experience increased thirst, so we'll be able to flush out the excess. Urination will increase, and sodium levels can drop. Here we need to balance and strengthen the Kidneys with formulas like Liu Wei Di Huang Wan, while addressing any associated Dampness, Phlegm, and Stasis.

Antidiabetic pharmaceuticals may be able to keep blood sugar levels in balance and prevent organ failure, but as usual they don't address the cause. It is easier for doctors to control blood sugar levels with these drugs without stressing the necessity of dietary adjustments, exercise, and stress reduction. Type I diabetes requires insulin administration in order for the cells to utilize glucose. In Type II diabetes, the cells have become resistant to insulin, but often this can be rectified through diet and lifestyle changes. Gestational diabetes can occur during pregnancy because of the increased demands of the Spleen, but usually resolves after childbirth. Obstetricians treat gestational diabetes like Type II diabetes, administering oral hypoglycemics. Dietary adjustments and supplements can often keep blood sugar levels within normal limits to stave off the need for pharmaceuticals. Alzheimer's disease has been described as Type III diabetes, as the brain becomes resistant to the effects of insulin. The plaque formations and neurofibrillary tangles found in the brains of Alzheimer's patients could be seen as equating to Phlegm accumulation and Blood stasis. Since diabetic patients have a higher likelihood of developing Alzheimer's disease, prevention is the best cure.

In all of these metabolic conditions, the Spleen is weakened, and the diet needs to be cleaned up to create an alkaline environment to resolve the inflammation. Dampness often won't be resolved until the Heat is cleared. Encourage the elimination of all added sugars and sweeteners, refined carbohydrates, alcohol, wheat, corn, dairy, and conventionally farmed meat and dairy products. Even caffeine can raise blood sugar by triggering the release of adrenaline, which tells the liver to release stored glucose. The anti-cancer or anti-inflammatory diets are good places to start. Suggest a menu plan consisting of organic vegetables, bitter greens, seeds, and nuts. Proteolytic enzymes can be added when the blood is alkaline enough. Supplements that help normalize blood sugar include berberine, chlorophyll, NAC, chromium picolinate, fenugreek, bitter melon, and inositol.

Antidiabetic drugs
Insulin
These preparations are administered in Type 1 diabetes, as the beta cells of the pancreas are unable to produce insulin. Without insulin, blood glucose continues to rise, potentially damaging the eyes, kidneys, and nerves. There are several types of insulin preparations on the market that vary in how quickly they act to control blood glucose and how long they can control blood sugar levels. Insulin breaks down through digestion, so insulin is delivered via injection, pen, or pump.

Rapid acting: regular insulin (Humulin R, Novolin R, Velosulin, Regular Iletin I), onset 30–60 minutes, duration 5–8 hours.

Prompt insulin zinc suspension, onset 1–2 hours, duration 12–16 hours. Lispro insulin solution (Humalog), onset 15 minutes, duration 6–8 hours.

Intermediate acting: insulin isophane (Humulin N, NPH-N, NPH Iletin,

Novolin N), onset 1–2 hours, duration 24–28 hours. Insulin zinc suspension (Humulin L, Lente Insulin, Lente Iletin I and II, Novolin L), onset 1–3 hours, duration 24–28 hours.

Long acting: extended insulin zinc suspension (Humulin U Ultralente), onset 4–8 hours, duration more than 36 hours.

The side effects of insulin include hypoglycemia, weight gain, and abnormal fat distribution. During hypoglycemic episodes, patients become lightheaded or dizzy and shaky, and they sweat and experience rapid heart rate, blurred vision, confusion, and tingling in the extremities. All of these effects are due to manipulating the transportation function of Spleen Yang and its effects on blood sugar.

Hypoglycemics

These are meant to be prescribed for those diagnosed with Type II diabetes, whose cells exhibit resistance to the effects of insulin, causing blood glucose to remain elevated. However, some of these drugs are prescribed in "pre-diabetic" scenarios, supposedly to curtail the development of diabetes. Most hypoglycemic medications are administered orally. Each, in its own way, will attempt to reduce blood glucose levels either by raising insulin release from the pancreas or attempting to force glucose into the cell, bypassing the body's strained Spleen Qi and Yang.

Sulfonylureas

- Tolbutamide (Orinase)
- Tolazamide (Tolinase)
- Acetohexamide (Dymelor)
- Chlorpropamide (Diabenese)

These drugs have two main mechanisms of action: they act on the pancreatic beta cells to stimulate insulin secretion, and they increase the sensitivity of tissues to the actions of insulin. Sulfonylureas bind to pancreatic beta cells' ATP-sensitive potassium channels, which alters their resting membrane potential, causing an influx of calcium which then stimulates the secretion of insulin. These drugs may cause hypoglycemia as they drive more glucose into the cells, thus lowering blood levels. In addition to causing low blood sugar, other side effects include increased hunger, stomach upset, and weight gain. They disrupt the dynamics of Spleen and Stomach Qi, and are usually not used alone anymore in the management of diabetes.

Second generation agents

- Glipizide (Glucotrol)
- Glyburide (Micronase, Diabeta)
- Gliclazide
- Glimepiride

These are more potent than sulfonyureas. The required dosage is lower than sulfonyureas, but their ability to control glucose isn't substantially higher. Adverse effects include syncope, dizziness, nervousness, anxiety, depression, hypoesthesia, insomnia, pain, paresthesia, drowsiness, headache, diaphoresis, pruritus, hypoglycemia, increased lactate dehydrogenase, diarrhea, flatulence, dyspepsia, and vomiting. Like the sulfonyureas, they overly stimulate and disrupt the Spleen and Stomach Qi and Yang. Counterflow may result from excess Yang stimulation, while the resulting fall in blood sugar may cause the Spleen Qi to crash.

Non-sulfonyureas
Biguanides

- Metformin (Fortamet, Glucophage, Glumetza, Glucovance, Glycon, Riomet)

These blood sugar modulators are used to treat Type II diabetes by enhancing the cells' sensitivity to insulin, increasing glucose uptake and utilization, without causing hypoglycemia. Metformin also reduces hepatic gluconeogenesis and decreases the intestinal absorption of glucose. A secondary benefit is that they can induce weight loss. Metformin also inhibits mitochondrial ATP and liver uptake of lactic acid, which can lead to serious lactic acidosis, especially in those with impaired renal function. Metformin can also cause deficiencies in vitamin B12. Side effects of the drug include nausea, vomiting, diarrhea, flatulence, loss of appetite, abdominal pain, chest discomfort, muscle pain, malaise, skin rash, flushing, palpitations, headaches, chest discomfort, chills, weakness, dizziness, and nail disease.

Inhibiting the production of glucose in the liver, its absorption in the intestines, and forcing glucose into the cell without increasing Spleen Yang can disrupt the ascending function of Spleen Qi, interfere with the Stomach Qi's descending function and intestinal mobility, obstruct Liver Qi, and lead to Liver-Spleen disharmony, Qi stagnation, and Yin deficiency. Patients often complain of the side effects, and it's important to know that metformin is not addressing the cause of glucose elevations and does not improve pancreatic function. When working with patients on metformin, tonify the Spleen Qi and Yang, reduce counterflow, regulate the ascending/descending dynamic, and harmonize Liver Qi.

Thiazolidinediones or glitazones

- Pioglitazone (Actos)
- Rosiglatazone (Avandia)

These increase insulin sensitivity and also bind to a nuclear receptor known as the peroxisome proliferator-activated receptor gamma (PPAR-γ) which raises adiponectin, increasing adipocytes' insulin sensitivity and stimulating fatty acid oxidation. Side effects include increased hunger, thirst, and urination, weight gain, edema, hypoglycemia, heart failure, headache, bone fractures, sinusitis, pharyngitis, visual changes, and flushed dry skin.

While glitazones ramp up the Spleen Yang's response to glucose, this unharmonized approach can also disrupt fluid metabolism, increase Stomach Fire, deplete Liver Yin and Blood, and cause Dampness. Our approach will be to tonify Spleen Qi, drain Dampness, and clear Stomach Fire. Because of their Heating effects, patients with pre-existing Yang Ming Heat might do better on metformin than Actos.

Glucagon-like peptide 1 (GLP-1)

- Semaglutides (Ozempic, Wegovy, Rybelsus, Trulicity, Victoza)
- Tirzepatide (Mounjaro)

These drugs are delivered by injection. Their effects mimic the actions of the gut hormone GLP-1, which is released in response to Gu Qi to prompt the pancreas to produce more insulin to reduce blood glucose levels. They also block the liver's release of glycogen, and are sometimes used to treat non-alcoholic fatty liver disease. This class of drugs has been growing in popularity as a weight loss drug, and many without diabetes are prescribed these pharmaceuticals to "prevent" the development of Type II diabetes without having to adjust their diet or lifestyle. The increased activity of GLP-1 sends signals to the brain that tell it the stomach is full, slowing down the metabolism and making one feel full longer, which is one of the reasons individuals lose weight while on them. When they stop taking these drugs, however, the weight they lost returns. Hence, many stay on them for life, which is always a boon for the industry. While there have been exploding sales of semaglutides, touted as the new wonder drug for weight loss as they supposedly reduce the risk of cardiovascular events due to obesity, they leave the gastrointestinal system with quite a few unfortunate side effects, including hypoglycemia, nausea, vomiting, flatulence, heartburn, constipation, and dry mouth. These drugs can also cause fatigue and actual muscle loss. More serious side effects include pancreatitis, visual changes, kidney issues, gallbladder problems, and thyroid tumors.

Patients are usually delighted with their new prescription, at least initially. As the drugs invigorate their Spleen Yang, they watch their excess weight come off. Yet there is always a price to pay. When Spleen Yang is overly focused on putting away sugar, other aspects of the Earth element may suffer. Spleen Qi decreases; Stomach Fire may increase, and despite the weight loss, their muscles often weaken and their energy levels suffer. Yang Ming is stifled, which can cause Heat and stagnation.

Eleanor had always been a bit "pudgy," and even though her blood sugar and hemoglobin A1C were within normal limits, her doctor prescribed Ozempic to help her lose weight. Within a few months, she lost over 40 pounds without even trying, and could fit into clothes she hadn't been able to squeeze into for many years. She was thrilled with the weight loss, and thought she had found the fountain of youth and beauty. Her stomach remained a bit upset, and she always had a stomach ache; she burped and had gas almost constantly, but she decided to focus her mind on her improvement, and considered them minor annoyances. She was tired all the time, and started to drink coffee throughout the day, even though it exacerbated her new symptom of heartburn. She also began to experience blurred vision, and had to get a new eyeglass prescription. Her hair was falling out at a rather alarming rate, and so her once long and thick hair was cut into a pixie. Next, she noticed that her face started sagging, her cheeks looked hollow, and there was a dramatic increase in the number of wrinkles around her eyes and mouth. She chocked it up to the weight loss, and went to a skin care clinic for dermatologic facial fillers. She also noticed how weak her muscles were becoming, and while her body was lighter according to the bathroom scale, it felt much heavier and more difficult to maneuver. Eventually she could hardly recognize herself anymore, which made her anxious and depressed, symptoms she had never experienced before. Her husband and kids were worried about her, too. As she began to contemplate all of these changes, she decided she didn't like who she was becoming, and that the weight loss wasn't worth the lost quality of life. Eventually she chose to stop getting the injections. Within a year she had regained most of the lost weight, and along with it she got her "dear pudgy self" back again.

Despite what the pharmacological research reports, interfering with metabolism is not an innocuous process. From the 1930s to the 1960s, drug studies showed that amphetamines were a great idea for weight loss, as well as reducing fatigue and lifting depression (Rasmussen, 2008). Considered safe, prescriptions were backed by the FDA and utilized and promoted in US military combat (Rasmussen, 2011). The side effects of semaglutides are due to the medicine's overstimulating effects on Spleen and Stomach Yang, causing counterflow and disrupting fluid metabolism, while simultaneously blocking the Qi of the Liver. Liver Yin and Blood deficiency may also result. Again, when Yang Ming Heat is present, the side effects will be worse.

Other categories of hypoglycemic pharmaceutical preparations include meglitinides (Repaglinide), dipeptidyl peptidase IV inhibitors (Sitagliptin), and alpha-glucosidase inhibitors (Acarbose).

In most cases, those who are compliant with diet, lifestyle, and herbal treatments should be able to stop these medications altogether, especially with the help of Chinese medicine. Tonifying Spleen Qi and Yang, resolving Dampness, clearing Stomach Fire, and tonifying deficient Yin help support their Zang Fu to return to a harmonized state. When the wasting and thirsting condition is due to Heat in Yang Ming, Bai Hu Tang can help diminish the Stomach Fire that is weakening the Spleen, causing the diabetic scenario. Shi Gao and Gan Cao are powerful herbs for treating diabetes, so if one is taking hypoglycemics along with Bai Hu Tang, the synergistic effect may make them become hypoglycemic. Ge Gen's ability to generate fluids can also have an antidiabetic effect, so if on hypoglycemics, dosing may need to be adjusted. For patients who remain on medication, watch for Heat that will continue to damage the Spleen.

CHAPTER 8

Lipid-Lowering Pharmaceuticals, Atherosclerosis, and Cardiovascular Drugs

While a faulty sugar metabolism may provide the initial conditions that set up inflammation, fat attempts to address the corrosive effects of inflammation on the vascular walls by blanketing the Heat with the Yin effects of cholesterol. When Yin is dried up, the body will often produce Dampness as a compensatory surrogate. Drastic attempts to reduce blood cholesterol levels without addressing the cause can result in increased Heat and inflammation, stagnation, and Yin deficiency.

The nature of fat

Our ancestors have genetically programmed our systems to be drawn to fatty foods. Fat is the best source of long-term fuel, making us feel full and satisfied. When we are relaxed and satiated, our body releases hormones that make us feel content. Fat doesn't have its own flavor; it's not pungent, sour, salty, sweet, or bitter. Being generally neutral in flavor, our taste buds don't recognize fat by itself. Fat provides a special texture in the mouth more than flavor, although fat is able to concentrate scents and flavors that are cooked in it, allowing them to linger in your mouth, giving food more fullness and depth. Fat-free diets have only contributed to metabolic problems. Foods in which natural fat has been removed seem to lack substance. They taste somehow insufficient, as if their very essence has been removed. The fat is often substituted with some sort of gum or starchy equivalent, which is no better for the Spleen and Stomach.

Fat is a dense, energetic constituent of the metabolic pathway, providing slower and more sustained energy than carbohydrates or proteins, and correlating with Yuan Qi. Lipids are also associated with Gao, the pasty globular aspect of Gao Huang or fatty membranes, and Ye, the oily substance necessary to produce hormones so that Jing can interact through the Blood. Adipose cells can accumulate anywhere in the body; usually approximately 90 percent is stored as subcutaneous fat, where San Jiao transmits Yuan Qi to the Cou Li space, or as visceral fat surrounding organs beneath the abdominal wall. White fat consists of large white lipid drops that accumulate from excess dietary calories and is typically stored in the belly, hips, and thighs. The cells of brown fat contain iron-rich mitochondria. Brown fat thus stores more energy, and is more Yang in nature than the white Yin fat.

Metabolism of dietary fat

The stomach breaks fat down into smaller droplet particles which enter the small intestine where they are emulsified by bile, a bitter, alkaline, and rich medium containing bile salts, bilirubin, cholesterol, fatty acids, lecithin, and minerals. Bile is produced by the liver in amounts up to one liter per day, and is stored in and released by the gallbladder. Bile salts emulsify fat so that pancreatic lipase can digest it into free fatty acids and monoglycerides, which can then pass through small intestine villi to enter into the lymphatic capillary system and travel through lymph, a component of Ying Qi.

Fats bind toxins and acids, which then need to be alkalinized and neutralized by minerals, so they can be processed and released by the San Jiao and Gallbladder. This is how Shao Yang participates in the circulation of Jin/Ye. The Gallbladder's extraordinary function of storing bile allows this essence to be emptied to supply the Extraordinary Meridians and marrow with the fat they need.

Types of fat

Dietary sugar is transformed into body fat, but dietary sources of fat are handled differently. Once the fats are digested, fatty acids go into the lymphatic system; some is used for energy, and some will be stored in lipid droplets within fat cells. Glycerol is bound with fatty acid molecules for storage. When fat is needed, bile salts reduce the surface tension of the stored triglycerides so that lipase can break it back down into fatty acid and glycerol. The fat that you eat impacts your cholesterol more than the cholesterol that you eat. Only about 20 percent of the population reacts to or needs to be concerned about the intake of dietary cholesterol; the nature of the fat consumed seems to be a much greater factor.

Unsaturated fats

These are liquid at room temperature, and are found mostly in plants like nuts, seeds, and vegetables.

- Trans fats are naturally found in small amounts in some meat and dairy, but are not associated with increased risk of cardiovascular disease. Yet when liquid vegetable oils are artificially hydrogenated to remain solid at room temperature, they become more stable; in fact, too stable, making them difficult to get rid of. The chemical alteration caused by hydrogenation produces toxic effects in the body like cellular stress and inflammation. They are unable to be processed by the liver, so they tend to build up and potentially cause fatty livers, increased LDL, and a greater risk of cardiovascular disease.

- Monounsaturated fats contain one carbon-carbon double bond and are found in olive and peanut oils, avocados, almonds, hazelnuts, pecans, pumpkin seeds, and sesame seeds. These fats can help reduce LDL levels in the bloodstream.

- Polyunsaturated fats (PUFAs) contain two or more carbon-carbon double bonds, and also help reduce blood levels of LDL. Polyunsaturated fats are usually considered "better" than saturated fats because they chelate and bind to other fats; yet this also makes them become reactive in the presence of Heat. In patients who exhibit signs like a rapid pulse and red tongue, indicative of Heat, expect PUFAs to become reactive. This process turns the fat into rancid and toxic trans fats, making it more difficult to detoxify. In the presence of a sluggish liver, these toxic fats then accumulate.

- Omega 3 fatty acids must be obtained through dietary sources, as your body can't make these triple fatty acids that are a crucial part of cellular membranes. Omega 3s help lower triglyceride levels, and it is helpful to raise the ratio of O3 to O6.
  - ALA (alpha lipoid acid from plant sources, has to be converted to EPA and DHA to be utilized): soybean, rapeseed and flaxseed oils, walnuts, chia seeds.
  - EPA (eicosapentaenoic acid, a signaling molecule that has a cooling effect in the Blood).
  - DHA (docosahexaenoic acid, vital for brain development, skin, and vision). These are found in fatty fish, some seafood, and algae.
- Omega 6 fatty acids are also essential to obtain from the diet. Omega 6s provide energy but are also inflammatory in higher quantities. Found in most vegetable oils such as safflower, sunflower, rapeseed, sesame seed oils, nuts, and seeds, many of these refined, industrial seed oils are heated to very high temperatures in order to oxidize the fatty acids. They are further highly processed by bleaching and deodorizing, creating toxic and pro-inflammatory by-products that are toxic to the body.

Saturated fats

The carbon atoms of these fats are saturated with hydrogen atoms, making them solid at room temperature. They are found mainly in animal sources like pork, beef, eggs, and dairy, but also in high levels in coconut and palm oil. Saturated fats have been viewed as unhealthy because they hang around in the body longer. Yet because they are more stable and non-reactive than unsaturated fats, they are not prone to breakdown and therefore will be a healthier Yin alternative for patients who exhibit signs of Heat.

Triglycerides compose about 95 percent of our dietary fat. They are formed from glycerol and three fatty acid molecules, both saturated and unsaturated. Unused calories are converted into triglycerides and stored in fat cells. As fat builds up, the body creates three glyceride receptors to bind the fat so it can circulate through the system. This conversion of fat into triglycerides occurs in the liver, and the breakdown of triglycerides also relates to the Lung's ability to diffuse, descend, and detoxify.

Elevated triglyceride levels may be associated with pancreatic (Spleen) dysfunction, hypothyroid, metabolic disorders, metabolic syndrome, liver disease, and heart attacks. Because triglycerides are made from sugar and fat, the patterns of impaired glucose metabolism (Spleen Yang/Qi deficiency) are pertinent here as well. Further, the Lung is the major organ to help the body get rid of fluids: externally via diffusion and sweating, while its descending function provides exit via urination and defecation; and via expectoration if there is Phlegm stagnation. As triglycerides build up, weak Lung Qi function can fail to flush out excess levels. This whole scenario represents a weakness of Spleen and Lung Qi, predisposing to an internal environment of Dampness, Damp Heat, or Phlegm, often complicated by Liver Qi stagnation. When triglycerides are high, it can impact oxygen and CO^2 levels. Palpate the Lung meridian and look for sensitivity around Lu 1, 7, and 9. Sometimes, temporary elevations in triglycerides can cause Lung congestion and coughing. Increasing dietary fiber and oatmeal can also help chelate excesses for the bowels to evacuate. Remember that our Lungs help us release sorrow, and if our emotions are stuck, our entire letting go mechanism might be impaired.

Normal blood levels of triglyceride are presently considered to be below 200 mg/dL, the optimum being 100. This norm is changing, however. While 250 used to be considered normal, the "new" normal is now less than 150 mg/dL, with 150–200 mg/dL considered borderline. According to the conventional medical approach, this means "treat with lipid-lowering pharmaceuticals."

Cholesterol

Because cholesterol is such a crucial substance, it is produced within the body. Over three-quarters of the body's cholesterol is engendered by the liver, while the remaining is derived from dietary sources. Cholesterol is considered a component of Jing and is foundational in the production of cellular membranes, hormones, and vitamin D.

Cholesterol is Yin and protects the body from Heat and Fire toxins. Oxidation puts out Heat, and cholesterol is a great antioxidant.

Optimum cholesterol values are said to be under 200 mg/dL; borderline levels are listed at 201–239; and high levels above 240 mg/dL. But, of course, we can't make such broad and sweeping generalizations. At times in life, our cholesterol values need to be higher. We take on more fat when we need greater protection. Ethnicity and geography also play a role, as those who hail from Western European countries tend to have higher cholesterol levels, while those from African countries are generally lower. According to a 2011 study published in *The Lancet* (Finucane *et al.*, 2011), the USA, Canada, and Sweden had relatively low cholesterol values. The study did not take into account dietary and lifestyle practices, or how many people were being treated with cholesterol-lowering drugs.

Integrated into the membrane for flexibility, cholesterol maintains the integrity and elasticity of cellular membranes by insulating them and protecting the Yuan Qi. Every seven or so years in a female or eight years in a male, the Yuan Qi exposes itself to work out any unresolved issues held in the Jing-Shen axis. During these transitional times, we often feel vulnerable and in need of extra protection. If the Heart is overly challenged during these times of psychic confrontation, cholesterol levels may rise to protect the organs from damage. Interestingly, later in life high cholesterol is associated with better cognitive function. The brain, or Sea of Marrow, is an extraordinary Fu, and when Jing declines, Yuan Shen no longer has the strength of substance to empower Shen Ming, the radiance of the Spirit, to shine.

Cholesterol is the precursor to active hormones. Active hormones occupy specific cellular receptors to exert their effects on the cell. The process by which cholesterol becomes the active hormone represents the junction between Yuan and Ying Qi levels, or the process by which Jing becomes Blood. We can view cholesterol as Liver Yin, or more specifically the pathway whereby Kidney Yin and Liver Yin, which share the same source, engender Liver Blood. The pathway where the active hormone estradiol (Liver Blood) is produced from cholesterol exemplifies this process through these intermediary steps: cholesterol ▸ pregnenolone ▸ dehydroepiandrosterone (DHEA) ▸

androstenedione ▶ estrone ▶ estradiol. Liver and Kidney Yin may also be transformed into Kidney Yang by a similar pathway where adrenal hormones and the active hormone testosterone are produced: cholesterol ▶ pregnenolone ▶ DHEA ▶ androstenedione ▶ testosterone. The different pathways cholesterol takes correlates with how our creative Yin and Yang energies express themselves. This includes different forms of hypercholesteremia as well. There are three different types of cholesterol, carried in lipoproteins which are made up of fats, proteins, and sugar, in varying degrees.

VLDL

These extremely light lipoproteins are derived from dietary fats and excess calories that are converted into triglycerides. The composition of very low density lipoproteins consists of about 90 percent lipid and 10 percent protein. VLDL levels estimate the percentage of triglycerides found in the body. High VLDL levels may represent patterns of Dampness or Damp Heat from an underlying Spleen Qi and Yang deficiency, or Lung Qi deficiency.

LDL

Low density lipoproteins are big and fluffy cholesterol molecules, and represent the mechanism whereby the Liver sends Yin out to the periphery to patch up endothelial walls that have been damaged by elevated pressure, heat, and oxidative damage (Heat, Qi stagnation, Depressive Heat, Liver Yang rising). While fat levels may be high for other reasons, this Yin mobilization is often a necessary response to inflammation; not necessarily a "cause" in and of itself. While Western medical standards always focus on lowering LDL, it is helpful to know that LDL is a Yin substance, which in excess can reduce blood flow through the vasculature. But elevated LDL levels are considered an effect, not a cause. High Blood levels of LDL may be associated with Spleen Qi and Yang deficiency, and the accumulation of Dampness and Phlegm. Larger LDL particles correlate with weakness of the Spleen Qi's ability to contain the size, resulting in more Dampness and Phlegm. However, systemic inflammation can be the cause of elevated LDL, where Damp accumulation is the compensation for Heat. In these cases, Heat must be remedied. Heat oxidizes LDLs (oxysterols), which can in turn become rancid, producing more Heat and Fire toxins, and then more LDL...

Finally, calcium may be called in to neutralize the acidity and cement any tears in the blood vessel walls, a process by which arterial plaques are formed that narrow the lumen of the Blood vessels. Now we have Heat, Damp, Phlegm, and Blood stasis. Elevations can be addressed with a stress-reducing lifestyle, clearing Stagnation, Heat, and Dampness and adopting a Mediterranean-type diet that includes lots of sour foods like lemon, artichokes, and olives, especially if the sides of the tongue are red and elevated and the left Guan pulse is wiry and rapid. Supplementing with red rice yeast extract can also help LDL levels.

Lipoprotein (a), a genetically determined variant of LDL, is produced by hepatocytes and is involved in wound healing and repair. Lp(a) elevations are considered an atherogenic risk factor in those with heart or vascular disease, atherosclerosis, and strokes. Blood tests aren't routinely ordered since Lp(a) levels aren't affected by statin drugs or dietary adjustments, although supplements like niacin and flaxseed can lower them. Even those with normal LDL levels can have elevations in Lp(a) (more than 30 mg/dL), which stimulates the release of clotting factors, binds to pro-inflammatory oxidized phospholipids, and competes with an enzyme that breaks down clots. Lp(a) levels indicate one's underlying propensity for Yin to be transformed, via Heat, into Phlegm through mechanisms that involve hypofunctioning of Spleen Qi and ascendant Yang. This dynamic is involved in the Yang pattern of hyperlipidemia, which will be described below.

HDL

High density lipoproteins are small carrier molecules produced by the Liver and Small Intestine that transport LDL and triglycerides back to the Liver and into the intestine for removal. HDL also helps deliver fat soluble nutrients and repairs damaged cells in the nervous system. It is basically a recycling mechanism for LDL.

Optimum levels of HDL are greater than 60 mg/dL, and ideally should be more than 40 percent of the total cholesterol count. Unexpectedly high HDL levels can be associated with heavy metals (excess Cold) or other toxic exposure. Low levels can be due to inflammation and androgens (Heat). Exercise, Mediterranean-type diets, fish oils, and niacin can help increase HDL levels. Thus, HDL levels can be seen as a measure of Yang mobilization and its ability to root back in the Lower Jiao.

Patterns of hyperlipidemia

Hypercholesterolemia tends to manifest as one of the two following scenarios: underlying Kidney and Liver Yin deficiency (they share the same source) with Yang excess (Heat, Damp Heat), or Spleen and Kidney Yang deficiency with Yin excess (Dampness). All can show up with Liver Qi stagnation, ascendant Yang, and Liver/Gallbladder Damp Heat.

In the excess Yang scenarios, we usually find that Yin is deficient, Heat is present, and lipids are rancid. Here we need to nourish Yin, perhaps with Zuo Gui Yin or Zhi Bai di Huang Wan, and clear Heat with fat-soluble antioxidants like vitamin E and A. These patients will benefit from non-reactive saturated fats like ghee, butter, and coconut oil.

In the excess Yin patterns, the patient has more Dampness (with underlying Spleen Qi deficiency), and antioxidants will only stagnate the Qi. They will do better with low fat diets, exercise, polyunsaturated fatty acids to facilitate metabolism of sterol lipids, green tea extract, digestive enzymes, and Omega 3 fatty acids.

Cholesterol increases in response to fungal infections, which are considered Damp. Aspirin, as we saw, invigorates the Blood and clears Dampness. As the Damp environment in which fungus thrives is resolved, the body doesn't need the increased cholesterol to address the inflammation.

Fat is first and foremost a Yin substance, necessary for cellular health, protection, neural signaling, hormonal processes, and energy production. Excess fat stores create a Damp environment, where Heat can spoil the fat to create toxicity. In a state of heated oxidation, there is an excess of electrons called free radicals which can cause major cellular damage to the body. Oxidation equates with Fire toxins, which increases catabolic activity, cellular breakdown, systemic inflammation, degeneration, and poor oxygenation of tissues. While fat fuels and protects, fat also holds toxins and maintains latency. So properly diagnosing the underlying patterns and treating their manifestations can resolve the justification for lipid-lowering drugs.

Lipid-lowering drugs
Bile-acid-binding resins

- Cholestyramine (Question, Prevalite)
- Colesevelam (Welchol)
- Colestipol (Colestid)

Bile acid sequestrates are administered to reduce LDL levels by binding to bile acids in the intestines, thus preventing the reabsorption of bound cholesterol into the body. This decreases bile acids, causing increased synthesis of bile acids from cholesterol in the liver. This also results in increased activity of LDL receptors, enhancing the removal of LDL from the bloodstream. Side effects of bile-acid-binding resins include constipation, stomach pain, vomiting, heartburn, gas, bloating, loss of appetite, fatigue, muscle aches and pains, gallstones, and weight loss. The binding effects that prevent reabsorption cause stagnation in the Small Intestine. This mechanism is responsible for the majority of the side effects, which can slow the absorption of food, and also lead to elevated triglyceride levels. There are likely to be underlying patterns of Damp Heat, and while superficial Dampness may be reduced by these drugs, the prolonged exposure to bile can create more Heat, resulting in inflammation and ulcers of the esophagus, stomach, and intestines. Small Intestine Heat can also transfer to the Urinary Bladder to cause symptoms of cystitis. Yang Ming Heat and Urinary Bladder Heat are thus common patterns brought about by bile-acid-binding resins.

Statins

- Atorvastatin (Lipitor)
- Fluvastatin (Lescol)
- Lovastatin (Mevacor, Altoprev)
- Pravastatin (Pravachol)
- Rosuvastatin calcium (Crestor)
- Siomvastatin (Zocor)

These statin drugs, prescribed to lower blood cholesterol values, are one of the most lucrative drugs produced by the pharmaceutical industry, with annual global sales reaching toward 20 billion dollars. You can see why the industry has little incentive to curtail their use. Lowering cholesterol and triglycerides through pharmaceutical means has become the goal rather than looking at the whole picture. Not everyone with elevated cholesterol is at risk for heart attacks.

The *British Medical Journal* published numerous articles in 2013 to question the narrative about fats and statins. In one (Abramson, 2013), it was stated that saturated fat is not the major issue, that fat-lowering diets have increased our cardiovascular risk, and the obsession with cholesterol levels has led to the "overmedication of millions of people with statins." Another (Malhotra, 2013) reported that statins were overprescribed to people with low risk of heart disease, and that the side effects caused more troublesome risk than the improvement in heart attack risk provided by the lipid-lowering drugs. And a third (Briggs, Mizdrak, & Scarborough, 2013) reported that an apple a day was as effective at keeping the doctor away than daily statin use. Of course, these studies have been criticized.

While statins do lower circulating levels of cholesterol in the blood, they have not been found to actually prevent heart attacks. Some doctors are now starting to limit recommending statins to patients who have been diagnosed with arterial plaques, heart disease, and those who have had heart attacks or strokes. But most physicians still prescribe solely based on blood cholesterol values. The atherosclerotic cardiovascular disease (ASCVD) risk score assesses percentage of estimated ten-year risk of having a cardiovascular incident. Assessment criteria are based on age, sex, race, blood pressure, LDL cholesterol levels, diabetes, hypertension, and smoking history. Values under 5 percent indicate low risk, whereas those over 20 percent indicate higher risk. In 2021, an article in the *BMJ Evidence-Based Medicine* (DuBroff, Malhotra, & de Lorgeril, 2021) evaluated drug trials to assess whether lowering total cholesterol and LDL cholesterol resulted in fewer cases of heart disease, and found there was no correlation.

Statins are suppressive in nature, blocking the liver's production of cholesterol, and causing the liver to remove cholesterol from the bloodstream. The mechanism by which they work is by blocking the liver's synthesis of cholesterol. This action obstructs Liver Yin by preventing Liver Blood's ability to nourish Kidney Yin. As statins remove cholesterol from the bloodstream, they address the manifestation of Dampness and Phlegm, but not the cause. The strong inhibitory effects can severely stagnate and burn out the Liver. Side effects include joint and muscle pain, digestive problems, mental fog, flu-like symptoms, skin rashes, hair loss, and sensations like pins and needles. They can also lead to the development of pancreatitis and hepatitis.

Cholesterol is protective and necessary for many essential body functions like hormone production. If cholesterol production is pharmacologically obstructed, the body will have to find other sources to create the Yin it needs. When Liver and Kidney Yin are depleted, sometimes the only way to compensate is by trying to build up and hold on to Lung Yin. Individuals may develop lipomas—Phlegm stasis that the body can't reabsorb—as fatty deposits show up within the Cou Li space. Heart Yin may also be diverted to support Kidney Yin, weakening the Heart and predisposing one to a higher risk of Heart disease. Blocking the Liver's production of cholesterol can also deplete the body's synthesis of natural antioxidants like Coenzyme Q10, and while cholesterol numbers may be reduced, tissue damage often continues to increase because free radicals produce Fire oxidation in the Blood. While statins may reduce the expression of Dampness and Phlegm as it relates to cholesterol levels in the blood, they do not fortify or invigorate the Spleen to resolve Dampness. They also stagnate Liver Blood. Blocking Liver Yin and depleting Liver Blood can give rise to Liver Qi stagnation and result-ing Heat. The Liver then can overact on the Spleen, further weakening its ability to resolve Dampness. The Yin and Blood blocking effects of statins also prevent full diastolic relaxation. Clearly, those with underlying Yin and Blood deficiency will experience fewer therapeutic and more troublesome side effects. Taking antioxidants, vitamin E, and Coenzyme Q10 can help reverse Heat-induced statin injury, as can treatments which fortify Liver Yin and Blood.

Use herbal formulas that regulate Qi, like Da Cheng Qi Tang and Xiao Chai Hu Tang, in order to regulate Blood, instead of Blood movers. Clear Liver Fire with herbs like Zhi Zi, Long Dan Cao, and Da Huang. Yin Chen Hao (Artemisia Capillaris) can protect the Liver from the toxicity of statins, but it may also slow down drug metabolism, which might increase the effects of the drug, making the patient feel even more uneasy. Milk thistle can also reduce the toxic effects on the Liver. In the Yin excess type of hyperlipidemia, statins will likely have more therapeutic effects than in the excess Yang type.

Atherosclerosis and cardiovascular drugs that invigorate the Blood

Atherosclerosis begins with inflammation which often results from an underlying deficiency of Yin, Yang, Qi, or Blood. The Qi stagnates, leading to depressive Heat, which then damages the intimal lining. And the Liver initiates the lipoproteins needed to cover it over. The Spleen also releases clotting factors in response to the break in the vascular wall. As LDL accumulates in the breach in the arterial walls, chemical changes signal endothelial cells to latch onto white blood cells. Wei Qi then penetrates the intima, causing a local Heat response. The inflammation transforms LDL into fat-laden foam cells, Phlegmy atherosclerotic plaques develop, and eventually they form fibrous caps, which turn into blood clots that can block the flow of blood to the heart, triggering heart attacks.

Thrombocytes or platelets are fragments of the blood-making megakaryocytes, which are manufactured in the bone marrow but stored in the Spleen, and represent how we hold on to our Blood. These non-nucleated discoid cells aggregate and connect to each other at sites of injured endothelium to curtail bleeding, not just by plugging up holes but also by releasing serotonin, which narrows arterioles to slow the flow of blood. (Perhaps this mechanism explains how Yunnan Bai Yao, whose hemostatic effect has been found to alter the release of platelets, also possesses a mood-enhancing effect, by its ability to astringe psychic leakage.) The way we hold on to the Blood represents how we carry aspects of our past identity around with us. The Kidney official's sense of security and trust in ourselves needs to pair with the Spleen, which banks our sense of self. Any breach in this system may lead to the Spleen overly attempting to hold things in place in order to protect our wounds and retain our precious emotions and memories. As we age and our Blood resources diminish, the body-mind puts more effort into holding on to the Blood, making it more prone to becoming thick and clotty. This is also one of the reasons the elderly population can be seen to be more "set in their ways," right about the time their memories start to fade.

Our treatments will be assessing underlying deficiencies in Qi, Blood, Yin, or Yang, and addressing any Heat, Qi stagnation, Dampness, Phlegm, and/or Blood stasis present. If Blood stasis is a prominent pattern and our Blood-invigorating treatment strategies are ineffective, add Yang tonics and moxibustion to help get the Blood moving. Dang Gui Si Ni San is helpful when Cold compounds the pattern. It is important to remember that we need Yang to move the Blood, but if we go beyond the Heart Blood's capacity to be moved, we risk depleting Yang and injuring Blood. Fish oil is a helpful supplement that nourishes the Jing and mildly invigorates the Blood.

Aspirin is derived from the bark of the willow tree, which grows in damp and swampy environments. It thus harbors antifungal and anti-cholesterol effects that can reduce turbidity and Phlegmy plaque formation. This is one of the reasons aspirin is prescribed to reduce clotting tendencies.

Antiplatelet medications like clopidogrel (Grepid, Plavix) prevent platelets from sticking together to form clots through a mechanism that diminishes the Spleen's ability to bank the Blood, which results in a Yang-invigorating effect. The main side effects are bleeding and bruisability, and thus these medications are contraindicated in patients with ulcers or bleeding disorders. Other side effects include stomach pain, heartburn, indigestion, and diarrhea, as their weakening effect on Spleen Qi, combined with their Heating effect, can aggravate the digestive tract.

Anticoagulants

- Rivaroxaban (Xarelto)
- Dabigatran (Pradaxa)
- Apixaban (Eliquis)
- Edoxaban (Lixiana)

These are chemical substances more commonly referred to as blood thinners that reduce coagulation of the blood, thus prolonging clotting time. Anticoagulant medications include vitamin K antagonists, direct oral anticoagulants (DOACs), and low molecular weight heparins (LMWHs). The drug heparin is prescribed to invigorate the Blood in those at risk for strokes or with heart conditions. The most commonly prescribed anticoagulant is warfarin, which is prescribed to address clotting disorders, atrial fibrillation, and to prevent clot formations. Side effects include prolonged bleeding, nosebleeds, bleeding from the gums, blood in the urine and stools, and severe bruisability. Warfarin is derived from hay mold and prevents the liver from utilizing vitamin K to produce clotting factors. The invigorating effects of Coumadin and heparin impact the Liver Blood and the intestines, resulting in gastrointestinal bleeding. They can also interfere with the absorption of vitamin D and lead to osteoporosis. Anticoagulants can overly disperse and injure the Blood, leading to Blood deficiency, especially in cases where the clotting tendency is due to Blood stasis from Blood deficiency. They can also injure the Kidney Yang, which we need to disperse Blood.

Many herbs and food substances have anticoagulant effects, even dried ginger. It is commonly believed that any Blood-invigorating herbs should be used cautiously when one is taking anticoagulants. This is true if patients have weakness in the Liver or intestines. If not, Blood-invigorating herbs may be prescribed if Blood stasis is a presenting pattern.

Our profession is well versed in the positive benefits of stress reduction, eating a healthy diet, exercising, and getting enough sleep, on which we educate our patients. Then, of course, we must address the patient's presenting pattern. When atherosclerotic plaques present with angina pectoris, we can consider prescribing styrax formulae, or we can add Ban Xia to address Phlegm, Ji Nei Jin to break down calcifications, and Nattokinase—an enzyme made from bacteria grown on soy that breaks down fibrinogen, digests clots, and reduces LDL cholesterol. Patients with elevated cholesterol can supplement with niacin, red rice yeast extract, policosanol, cholestyramine, and bile-acid-binding resins.

Finally, we must ask if we have reached the root. After diet and lifestyle issues have been addressed and we have administered our Heat-clearing, Phlegm-resolving, Blood-moving treatments, we have to acknowledge that we are still in problem-fixing mode, which is considered low grade medicine. Are we able to move deeper and help to awaken the Fire of the patient's own Heart? While this level of work doesn't replace our mastery with acupuncture and herbs, it adds another dimension where, rooted in spirit, Shen can ignite an inner healing force to course through and produce most radical healing effects.

Mary Katherine, a 68-year-old overweight woman, came to the clinic on ten different medications including Levoxyl, Metopropolol, iron, metformin, Allegra, Fosamax, Activella, omeprazole, acetaminophen, and Lipitor. Previously diagnosed with osteoarthritis and seasonal allergies in the spring, she took her medicines all year round. As part of her "health care regimen," once a week she dutifully distributed her drugs in her pill box, and took them religiously on the appropriate day. Her medical history showed she had never fitted the criteria for anemia, hypertension, diabetes, or hypercholesterolemia. The prescriptions were reportedly "preventing" the development of these conditions, and the proton pump inhibitor was "protecting her stomach lining" from the effects of Tylenol. She felt tired, achy, bloated, and unwell overall. Her Spleen Qi was weak, resulting in Dampness, and her Liver Qi was very stagnant. She reported being exhausted all of the time and didn't have the energy or motivation to do what she loved most, which was to create art. She had just moved, she lived alone, and had few friends. She spent most of her time reading her iPhone, even during her treatments. Her diet consisted of lots of comfort food, most of which contained refined carbohydrates, and she watched TV a lot, because she hated the quiet which magnified her loneliness. In addition to tonifying her Spleen, draining Dampness, and harmonizing her Liver, part of her therapy was to fast from sugar and refined carbohydrates, and join an art class to reignite her passion and meet new people. Eventually, she became the president of her homeowners' association. Within a year, she was a different person. She lost weight, had a community of friends, was painting again, and was no longer plagued by loneliness or the effects of her pharmaceuticals. This is what it looks like when we treat people rather than their diseases.

CHAPTER 9

Endocrine and Hormone Modulators

The endocrine system isn't an isolated system per se, but a whole complex collaboration of glandular responses within which hormones are produced that regulate growth, development, metabolism, mood, sleep, and reproduction. The word endocrine refers to the process of internal secretions, and hormone means a vital principle which sets in motion certain instinctual activities. Hormones are therefore more like verbs—processes—than nouns or things. The entire functioning of the endocrine system represents how each life is harmonized within the rhythms of nature, as infinite ongoing micro-adjustments of glandular output keep us in synch with our environment. The amounts of hormones circulating in the blood are considered effects, not causes, where ongoing internal feedback regulates influx and outflow. Therefore, trying to adjust their levels through hormonal manipulation never reaches the root, but only confuses the self-regulating system.

Our unique biorhythms are established as our energy is distributed to respond to each moment, unique to each person's constitutional and temperamental makeup. From these micro-adjustments we also respond to the cyclical natures of the horary clock, day and night, the tidal pulls of lunar phases, and seasonal changes. It's really a bit shocking to think how prescribing hormones could ever attempt to control the delicate hormonal rhythms without supporting patients to adjust to and flow with the rhythms of their lives. Chinese medicine doesn't have a concept of the endocrine system per se, but hormonal communication could be equated with Blood and Qi circulation via the Jing Luo, or fluids by way of the San Jiao network. While the thin fluids of Jin correlate more to the exocrine system, the thick Ye fluids circulate as internal hormonal secretions, and are distributed by the Small Intestine, which receives the wisdom of the Heart and plunges it into the belly. The endocrine system primarily follows the Sheng cycle, yet gynecology also obeys the reverse Sheng flow, as its laws are governed by pre-Heaven.

Our endocrine systems may also be challenged by transitions involved in larger rites of passage as we move from one phase of life to another through cycles of seven or eight years. Our hormones are meant to be reset during these transformative periods, and one shouldn't expect them to remain consistent with externally established "norms." These cycles of life and the transformations contained within are governed by three innate forces of the First Ancestry of the Eight Extraordinary Meridians.

> The Tao gives birth to One; the One gives birth to Two;
> the Two give birth to Three; and the Three give rise to the ten thousand things.

- The first is union. Being Yin, unitive actions belong to Ren Mai, which illustrates the dynamic by which opposing forces like egg and sperm fuse together to bring us into being.
- The second is separation, a Yang function governed by Du Mai through which output from organs like the adrenal glands takes us into seeming division.
- The third, Chong Mai, integrates the first and second and resolves conflicts held in the two. As it governs transitions and makes adjustments between Yin and Yang, it gives rise to specific metabolic functions like thyroid output.

These three functions then express themselves through the other five Extraordinary Meridians, and also impact the Zang Fu.

The endocrine system doesn't function independently as its functions interface with all other systems, sensations, and states of mind; hence glandular output could be referred to as psycho-neuro-skeletal-gastro-immuno-hepato-renal-respiratory endocrinology. Add any other system I may have left out.

Hormonal output and circulation, the harmonizing process that follows the Sheng cycle, equilibrates the Curious Organs with the Eight Extraordinary Vessels, the Zang Fu, and our emotional response to the environment, all while maintaining the remarkable capacity to reproduce ourselves in the process. Hormonal harmonization represents our internal flexibility, resiliency, and ability to adapt; any amount of resistance, internal rebellion, or expecting life to be different from what it is can produce glandular imbalances of underproduction, overproduction, or stagnancy in flow. It is very important to understand that endocrine glands synchronize the body with external and internal factors via negative feedback. When the upper control centers in the brain trigger the gland below to release hormones, the presence of the hormone in the blood acts on target tissues and also mists upward to reduce the signaling factors produced by the hypothalamus and pituitary glands. This then reduces stimulation of the gland, momentarily ceasing hormonal output. Thus, they have a built-in regulatory system to maintain harmony. This equilibrium can be disrupted via emotional and climatic factors, and by any type of hormone replacement, whether bio-identical or synthetic. Once an exogenous hormone enters the bloodstream, the delicate adaptive synchrony of the pathway is interrupted. Pharmaceutical hormones don't cure hormonal imbalances; they override the imbalance. For example, once an individual is prescribed thyroid hormone, the thyroid gland can relax its production of T4 and essentially go to sleep, as the upper control centers perceive constant hormonal input in the blood and thus turn off thyroid-releasing and thyroid-stimulating hormones from the hypothalamus and pituitary gland in turn. The body then loses its ability to make micro-adjustments in output as environmental conditions and situations might dictate.

I have covered the interworking of the endocrine system in my book *The Spirit of the Blood* and other works, yet I feel it must be restated before we can fully understand how endogenous hormonal administration impacts the entire web of connectivity.

Hypothalamus—the center control seat

The pineal gland responds to darkness and light by producing Yin melatonin and Yang serotonin. Dubbed the "seat of the soul" by Rene Descartes, it sits behind and transmits impulses to the hypothalamus, a walnut-sized gland at the base of the brain which also receives hormonal input from all of the endocrine glands it regulates. The hypothalamus further assesses our sensory perception of the world, our emotional response to it, and then duplicates our mind into body chemicals. From this complex mingling of forces, it creates its own hormones to communicate with its minister, the pituitary gland. The hypothalamus, like the Chong Mai, with its extraordinary capacity for adaptation, has an ancient evolutionary history, giving humanity the remarkable ability to respond to environmental stimuli through our deepest subconscious reactions.

Deep in the center of the brain, invisible sensory antennae pick up signals from without and within and convert them into currents of Qi. The hypothalamic's Qi impulses will then be translated by the pituitary gland into regulatory hormones, setting off the cascade of thick fluids that course through the waterways. The hypothalamus controls, among many other functions, the onset of puberty and regulation of the monthly ovulatory cycle as it also interfaces with the reverse Sheng cycle of gynecology. The hypothalamus releases somatostatin and dopamine, as well as thyrotrophin, corticotrophin, gonadotropin, and growth hormone releasing hormones. These releasing hormones direct the pituitary gland to produce the hormones that will stimulate each gland to emit their specific hormones into the blood, which will then act on the cells.

The Lungs direct the Qi, and allow letting go so that new possibilities can come into being. The Lungs also govern the corporeal soul, which oversees autonomic functioning, and the seven Po, which communicate in body sensations and moods that carry our soul's most treasured "issues," the gnarly lessons of life we are challenged to overcome. Interestingly, the entire endocrine symphony begins behind the nose, an area governed by Metal (Lung and Large Intestine). Primitive nose cells in the embryo secrete gonadotropin-releasing hormone (GnRH), which the other hormones follow. As the embryo develops, these GnRH secreting cells migrate to their final destination at the base of the brain that serves as the intersection between the nervous and endocrine systems, the junction of pain and pleasure. Smell is our most instinctive sense; when women are not inebriated or taking exogenous hormones like those found in hormonal birth control, studies have shown they can sniff out the sweat of men with whom their fertility is most compatible. Women who were drinking alcohol or had been prescribed hormonal birth control did not have access to this instinctual guidance.

We acclimate to our environment primarily by light, smell, and temperature. The Lung, which governs the left cerebral hemisphere, and the Liver, which governs the right, mark the passage of time—past and future—and between them, the empty center governed by the Earth element allows them to communicate through the thoroughfare of the corpus callosum fibers. Similarly, the hypothalamus occupies a center role where hormonal impulses blend together with other sensory and emotional input to direct output downstream.

We can liken the function of the hypothalamus as the regulatory center where Earth ascends to Metal to the dynamics of the Central Treasury at Lu 1 lifting to Lu 2 Cloud Gate. If our resonance with the macrocosm is ever lost, this is the place heavenly Qi can enter to restore our connection with the Source and re-establish this equilibrium throughout the kingdom. While all points on the body can feed back to impact the hypothalamus, direct points are located at Du 16, Du 17, and UB 10.

Primary hypothalamic dysfunction is addressed with the Eight Extraordinary Meridians.

Pituitary gland

Despite its small size tucked within a cavern of the sphenoid bone, the pituitary gland basically directs the entire Jing-Shen axis; supported, of course, by incoming information from the hypothalamus. Its little lookout point allows us to survey our inner landscape, reflect on our lives, and recognize all of the incoming and outgoing messages that create meaning in our lives. When we are lost in the Po's instinctive drives and consumed by subconscious moods, we tend to contract in fear and lose our larger and more panoramic perspective of life. Yet the Jing-Shen axis wants us to return back to the center into conscious influences carried in the Heart and Blood. Here we must make sure the Hun are rooted in the Liver and are able to commune with the Po in order to overcome our inner conflicts and thereby find completion within our lives. The inner channel of the Liver ascends along the neck, throat, nasopharynx, and eye and eventually terminates at Du 20, San Jiao's divergent link to the cosmos. The *Ode to Elucidate Mysteries* says, "Heaven, Earth, and human are the three powers. Baihui Du 20 echoes Heaven." Earth is reflected around the navel, and humanity in the Heart.

The Hun reside in the eyes by day, when they open up to project the world we see outside, and they rest in the Liver at night, where they penetrate the dream realm and leave the body through the portal at Du 20. There are three Hun (Dark Essence, Brilliance of the Fetus, and Clear Spiritual Force) that engage with the seven Po, provide guidance from the dream state, and create images to guide us on our journey. The Hun follow the Shen, and every two months the Hun report our progress to the Heavenly Emperor, and return with lessons or clues to support us on our journey. The complex function of the pituitary gland partly belongs to the Hun; in fact, the Hun regulate the functioning of the pineal, hypothalamus, and pituitary triad—where darkness becomes light, light becomes images, and images become not only our perceived reality, but the regulatory molecules that guide our decisions and movements. Our interpreted worldview manifests as pituitary hormones that shower forth to direct the rest of the endocrine symphony. As we become able to still the mind and gain access to the subtle pre-heavenly realms, we can pick up clues to the unfolding path of our soul's destiny. The more conscious we become of our internal patterns, the smoother our hormones are allowed to flow. So you can see how important it is to keep these pathways open as we follow the internal dictates to ascend to ever higher expressions of our destiny.

The posterior pituitary gland stores and releases hormones produced in the hypothalamus that pertain to the Heart-Kidney axis:

- Anti-diuretic hormone (ADH or vasopressin), which acts in the kidneys to regulate vasoconstriction, complex multi-cellular responses, social behavior, penile erection, response to testosterone, and male bonding. Its function equates with the dynamics of both Kidney Qi and San Jiao's regulation of body fluids.

- Oxytocin, a peptide hormone released in response to love and labor, which contracts the uterus, stimulates milk production in the breasts, along with chemicals that reduce stress and promote bonding in women. We can view its function as corresponding to the Fire officials Pericardium and San Jiao in promoting interconnectedness.

The intermediate pituitary cells produce melanocyte-stimulating hormones, which stimulate cells in the skin to produce melanin. Skin coloration, while expressed on the surface, belongs to Yuan Qi.

The anterior pituitary hormones include the following:

- Growth hormone (GH) regulates growth, metabolism, and body composition. Growth hormone is associated with production and distribution of Kidney Jing. Levels of growth hormone diminish as one ages, along with the ability to produce abundant Qi and Blood. Human growth hormone (HGH) supplements are like Jing, Qi, and Blood tonics on steroids. While they can promote strength and muscle growth in those with growth hormone deficits, taking exogenous HGH also can cause aches, pains, carpal tunnel syndrome, Type II diabetes, swelling, and gynecomastia, and create an increased risk of developing certain types of cancers.

- Adrenocorticotropic hormone (ACTH) stimulates the adrenal gland to secrete steroid hormones like cortisol, thereby regulating Kidney Yang.

- Prolactin (PRL) stimulates lactation milk production in the breasts. After delivery, the Blood lifts to the breasts, where it is released as milk, a function which correlates with the Small Intestine's role in supporting lactation. Prolactin elevations often correlate with Liver Qi stagnation and Damp Heat.

- Thyroid-stimulating hormone (TSH) stimulates the thyroid gland to secrete the Yang thyroid hormones. The pituitary gland responds to circulating thyroid hormone levels in the blood and hypothalamic release of thyrotropin, and releases appropriate levels of TSH in order to maintain metabolic equilibrium.

- Follicle-stimulating hormone (FSH) represents the Yang surge from above, which stimulates the gonads to produce eggs, sperm, and the active sex hormones estrogen and testosterone.

- Luteinizing hormone (LH) triggers ovulation and progesterone production in the ovary; it also stimulates testosterone production by the Leydig cells of the testes. In females, this hormone is released when Heart Blood, through the Pericardium, shifts its energies to the Liver, so has a strong Jue Yin association.

Pituitary hormone dysregulation often correlates with the pattern of Liver Qi stagnation, as a primary role of the liver is to metabolize hormones. If the liver doesn't have the strength to metabolize our own hormones properly, exogenous hormone administration further burdens the Qi, and strains inadequate Liver Blood. Most pituitary hormone abnormalities are resolved by addressing the system of dysfunction downstream.

I once worked with a woman who had a pituitary tumor that had ruptured, after which her adrenal glands, thyroid, and ovaries ceased to function correctly. In addition, she was diagnosed with diabetes insipidus, and had been prescribed cortisol, thyroxine, and estrogen, yet was constantly fatigued and foggy with persistent headaches. She had been to numerous specialists throughout the world, but this provided no relief, despite the many fasts, detox diets, and homeopathic, herbal, nutritional, and pharmaceutical remedies she had been prescribed. Her Liver Qi was somewhat stagnant, her Liver Blood and Spleen Qi were quite deficient, her system was very Damp, and she exhibited a classic Chong Mai imbalance. I prescribed a herbal formula with Spleen Qi tonics, herbs to invigorate the Spleen to resolve Dampness, Blood tonics, Qi harmonizers, and Kidney astringents. Treatments remained focused on the first and second trajectories of the Chong Mai as we delved into the shadow realm. In spite of the fact that she was a highly skilled spiritual teacher, there were still some blind spots where unexamined Po, lurking in the dark, begged to come out of hiding to communicate with the conscious realm. Her spirit was highly developed, but her humanity had been sorely neglected; a scenario which unfortunately is not uncommon in the healing realm. While it was difficult and intense work, within three weeks her energy was back, her headaches were gone, and she began slowly weaning off the hormones she had been taking for four years.

Corticosteroids are covered in the chapter on pain relievers.

Thyroid circuitry

The thyroid gland regulates metabolism and energy utilization and maintains the integrity of the skin. Similar to the function of Wei Qi, the thyroid hormone circulates warmth through the surface, and regulates the amount of calcium going to the muscles, nerve transmission, and peristaltic activity.

Nestled between Ren 22, Ren 23, and St 9, the butterfly-shaped thyroid gland takes its cues from how we respond to our environment via the negative feedback received from the upper centers, to determine how much Yang stimulation is required to meet the cellular requirements throughout the entire body. The Heart steams up the Celestial Chimney at Ren 22 to release the thyroid's warming, protective, and energizing functions, as its wings at St 9 Human's Welcome can be seen as fanning the release of hormones that regulate metabolism through protein synthesis, glucose utilization, and oxygen consumption. Thyroid hormone also regulates growth and tissue differentiation in the bones, muscles, and nerve cells, as well as assisting in digestive peristalsis and reproductive functioning.

Thus, the thyroid hormone represents certain aspects of Spleen and Stomach Qi and Heart Blood while mediating the Kidney Yin and Yang functions of gonadal and adrenal activity. Thyroid dynamics relate to how we express our creative passions in life. If we are lacking inspiration or our creative outlets are stifled, Yang may be inhibited as well. When the demands of our lives exceed Yang's capacity to keep up, the thyroid hormone may become overly taxed and plummet until conditions allow appropriate restoration. If, however, one gets blood work taken during periods of stress when thyroxine levels are not in the "normal" range, doctors are expected to prescribe a hormonal substitute. Thyroid abnormalities have become so commonplace these days that dysregulation is just expected and patients are automatically placed on medication.

Many years ago, the *Da Dai Li Ji* warned us that our modern tendency to be overly busy makes us become emaciated and miserable. Even more true today, the thyroid gland's primary failure stems from our fast-paced lives that exceed our ability to restore our Blood and Qi, and stress that congests the Qi of the Liver, producing stagnant environments that give rise to Heat that burns out our resources. Thyroid function may also become compromised by deficiencies of iodine, B vitamins, selenium, other minerals, antioxidants, and excess fluoride. I always recommend starting with the root, supplement deficiencies, and only considering medicating as a last resort. Symptoms of thyroid hormone deficiency include fatigue, feeling cold, weakness, dry skin, hair loss, weight gain, and constipation. This impaired metabolism is associated with Kidney Yang, Spleen Qi, and Blood deficiency. The proper functioning of the thyroid hormone relies heavily on the liver's ability to process the conversion of the storage form to the active hormone.

As universal intelligence converts light into water at the center of the brain behind the bridge of the nose, a stream of information flows down the throat to the neck area where the V of the Windows of Heaven conveys messages from the brain to the Heart and gut via the vagus nerve. Here, vibrations are transmitted outwardly through the larynx, and inwardly as our ability to listen deeply to our own intuitive guidance within is received by the Heart. This energetic vortex can direct us into our head and into our heart. The throat carries a unique dynamic at the root of the tongue, the chimney of the Heart. If you quiet your mind, you can notice that, as thoughts take shape as words, subtle muscular movements occur at the base of your tongue where the truth of the Heart is received via Jue Yin, and is either spoken or swallowed. Some conditions of thyroiditis have been linked to those who haven't been able to find their true voice, or haven't been able to articulate what they want in their lives. Those with overly busy minds might try calming this area to quiet the mind and tune into deeper guidance.

There is a complex circuitry through which piezoelectric impulses from the pineal gland, circulating thyroid hormone, and complex signals throughout the mind and body are conveyed to the hypothalamus, which responds by producing and distributing thyrotropin releasing hormone. This creates signals that are transmitted to the neighboring pituitary gland, which triggers the release of thyroid-stimulating hormone (TSH), whose normal ranges span from 0.5 to 5.0 mIU/L; this flows down to the thyroid gland to tell it how much thyroxine (T4) to release into circulation. The optimal functional range of TSH is 0.3–2.0. Low levels indicate adequate thyroid hormone (T4 and T3) in the blood; high TSH values indicate low thyroid hormone, and the pituitary gland has to make more thyroid-stimulating hormone to try to get the thyroid gland to work harder. As T3 and T4 hormone levels rise, TSH lowers, and vice versa. If T3 and T4 levels are normal but the tissues don't respond adequately, TSH will often be elevated. Giving more thyroid hormone won't make the body more responsive.

Thyroxine, T4, represents the Yin storage form of thyroid hormone. It is composed of four atoms of iodine attached to a tyrosine molecule, the precursor to norepinephrine and dopamine, which both act on the Heart. Iodine is a halogen, which holds heat, and is associated with the Spleen's banking ability. T4 is less Yang activating and more nourishing, functioning somewhat like Gui Pi Tang in its ability to nourish Spleen Qi and Heart Blood. Normal T4 levels should range between 5.0 and 12.0 mg/dL. Low levels of T4 might indicate Spleen Qi and Heart Blood deficiency; high levels are most often associated with Heart Yin deficiency or Heart Fire, among other individual patterns that will need to be resolved before the thyroid axis normalizes.

T3, tri-iodothyroxine, the more active form of thyroid hormone, is also produced in the thyroid gland, but it is converted from its inactive T4 form in cells from other body tissues by a process called deiodination, where one iodine atom is removed. It now becomes a more active molecule with only three heat-absorbing iodine atoms attached to the tyrosine molecule, rendering it more Yang and unstable. Normal T3 levels should range between 100 and 200 ng/dL, but most of our T3 is in the peripheral tissues, so blood levels can be misleading. Most of the conversion from T4 to T3 occurs in the liver. Thus, if the Liver Blood is deficient or its Qi stagnant, thyroid hormone levels may be adequate, but remain relatively inactive, as conversion to the active form is inhibited. T4's conversion to T3 is measured by Reverse T3, which should remain under 300 pg/dL. High levels of Reverse T3 are associated with Cold, deficient Yang, or stagnant Liver Qi. The active free T3 averages about 5 pmol/L. Low T3 can be associated with almost any deficiency in Qi, Blood, Yin, or Yang. If T4 is normal and T3 is low, look for signs of Liver Qi stagnation.

Hypothyroidism, which is diagnosed by elevated TSH values along with low T4 and/or T3 levels, can be associated with poor nutrition, inflammation of the thyroid gland, autoimmune thyroiditis, and cirrhosis, as well as other endocrine imbalances. Thyroid abnormalities are very common today; not only because we don't listen to our inner voices and respond adequately to environmental cues, but our soil has become mineral poor. Even Sun Simiao suggested that people who lived in the mountains far away from the sea consume sheep thyroid glands. Sea vegetables can help increase iodine levels as can applying topical iodine to the skin. A two-by-two-inch strip of Lugol's iodine solution on the inner arm should be absorbed slowly over a 24-hour period. If it disappears after a couple of hours, the rapid rate of absorption indicates that the body needs more iodine. Just reapply; the test is both diagnostic and therapeutic.

Hyperthyroidism is diagnosed when T3 and/or T4 are elevated; TSH will be normal or low. This condition often manifests with patterns of excess Yang like Liver and Heart Fire, and stirring of Wind.

Thyroglobulin antibodies (TgAb) should remain less than 20 IU/mL. Thyroid peroxidase (TPO) is an enzyme produced by the thyroid gland to manufacture thyroid hormone. The presence of antibodies to TPO (TPOAb) indicates that the immune system has identified the thyroid gland as foreign or threatening, perhaps because of underlying inflammation, and is mounting a response against it. These may present with conditions associated with abnormal blood sugar fluctuations such as diabetes or polycystic ovary syndrome. TPOAb can also be a marker of subclinical thyroid disease, which may manifest later as clinical symptoms associated with Hashimoto's thyroiditis or Graves' disease. Like many autoimmune disorders, the attack may stem from some type of emotional trauma—even very early in life—that has stressed the system, in this case the primary gland responsible for energy production. As repressed emotions lie dormant, pent-up anger, sorrow, or self-denial can build up enough pressure until the immune system, which assesses who is friend and who is foe, forgets its job and turns against itself, attacking its very source of vitality. This process was recognized in Japanese monks in the last century, who, while able to retreat from the world, couldn't escape from themselves or their internal issues. The high percentage of monks who developed autoimmune thyroiditis was theorized to have been caused at least in part by emotional suppression. Ongoing emotional suppression can unconsciously cause excessive defensiveness, which can stagnate or knot the Qi, and disarm the immune system, which forgets the identity it is supposed to protect and attacks with as much armature as Wei Qi can muster.

We can view the diagnosis of Hashimoto's thyroiditis as a breach in the body's boundaries, causing the immune system to become auto-reactive. The B and T cells become confused, and instead of deactivating foreign invaders, they turn against the thyroid cells that are supposed to be maintaining the very boundaries they are protecting. The overactive immune cells attack and kill thyroid cells, which then can no longer produce adequate quantities of thyroid hormone, resulting in hypothyroidism. The thyroid's Yang impulses can no longer support the body's metabolic demands, and victims experience the resulting deficiency symptoms of lethargy, depression, weight gain, dry skin, hair loss, constipation, and cold intolerance. Thyroid antibodies will be present, TSH will be elevated, and thyroid hormone reduced. The patient's underlying deficiencies of Yin, Yang, Qi, or Blood will need to be supplemented, and you will also need to reduce whatever excess (usually Heat and/ or Qi stagnation) might be presenting. The pulses may reveal weaknesses in the Spleen, Lung, or Heart energies, where Bu Zhong Yi Qi Tang or Gui Pi Tang would be appropriate; perhaps with Liver Qi stagnation, Xiao Yao San might be more fitting. Kidney Yang may need to be tonified with formulas like Jin Gui Shen Qi Wan. Generally, though, the best results can be obtained when you can accurately identify individual nuances in order to create a specific formula to modify the individual's unique internal landscape. Bu Zhong Yi Qi Tang might be modified by adding Du Zhong and Yin Yang Huo to tonify Kidney Yang.

Graves' disease is another autoimmune reaction against the thyroid gland. In contrast with Hashimoto's thyroiditis, where hypothyroidism results, in Graves' disease, the B and T cells of the immune system agitate the thyroid cells, making them overreactive, resulting in hyperthyroidism, with excess thyroid hormone production. This excess Yang presentation causes heart palpitations, nervousness, insomnia, fatigue, increased bowel movements, sweating, and heat intolerance. And when Yang becomes hyperactive, the body compensates by trying to slow it down; in this case with Phlegm production in the thyroid gland, which may become enlarged into a goiter. The patterns associated with goiter formation also involve Qi stagnation, when the size fluctuates along with emotional variations, and Blood stasis, when the goiter is fixed, hard, and painful. Further, Phlegm Heat mists the eyes, causing inflammation, cellular proliferation, and accumulation of fluid in tissues surrounding the eyeball, resulting in a condition called exophthalmos where the eyes bulge out. Patterns thus may include Liver Qi stagnation, Heat, Fire, and Phlegm congelation where turbid Yin cannot descend. We may regulate Qi, soothe the Liver, clear Heat and Fire, and resolve Phlegm with Lv 2, Lv 3, Pc 6, St 40, Ren 12, GB 1, GB 14, St 1, and Ll 4. Local points to address the goiter might include Ren 22, Ren 23, St 9, St 10, St 11, Ll 17, Ll 18, Sl 16, Sl 17, SJ 13, and Ping Ying, Shang Tian Zhu, and Hua Tuo Jia Ji of T1 and T2. Herbal formulations will of course need to address the presenting pattern, while adding herbs to soften (Kun Bo, Hai Zao, Xia Ku Cao, etc.) and dissolve the mass (Bie Jia, Mu Li, E Zhu, San Leng, Tu Bie Chong).

When thyroid imbalances are first identified, removing fluoride, and ensuring that adequate amounts of iodine, selenium, minerals, and antioxidants are present, while addressing the presenting patterns and causative lifestyle factors in most cases, can restore normal thyroid function without having to resort to medication.

The typical biomedical approach is to test TSH, T3, and T4 levels. If TSH is high, and/or thyroid hormone is low, a synthetic form of T4 is usually prescribed. Thyroxine is the preferred medication because it is more stable and easier to dose than T3. However, if the patient has patterns of Liver Blood deficiency or Liver Qi stagnation, adding more T4 to the system will not necessarily improve their condition, as the conversion to the active T3 form will still be impaired, and Yang stimulation will suffer.

When thyroid medication is prescribed, the thyroid gland no longer has to work to produce thyroid hormone. The hypothalamus and pituitary gland then sense adequate amounts of circulating thyroid hormone and turn down thyrotropin releasing hormone from the hypothalamus and thyroid releasing hormone from the pituitary gland; essentially putting the thyroid gland to sleep, as it no longer has a job to do. The longer a person is on thyroid hormone, the more likely it is that they will have to remain on it as it becomes difficult to wake up the thyroid gland after too many months or years of inactivity.

Thyroid hormone preparations

Thyroxine T4: Levothyroxine (Synthroid, Euthyrox, Levoxyl, Thyquidity, Unithroid). L-thyroxine is prescribed for diagnoses of hypothyroidism, and even in "subclinical hypothyroidism" which is a misnomer, because T4 levels are within normal limits, and patients are generally asymptomatic. This is usually a conversion problem, where Liver Qi stagnation is preventing the deiodination of the T4 storage form into the T3 active form, but many physicians prescribe L-thyroxine anyway, to "prevent" clinical hypothyroidism from manifesting. And of course, most patients comply. Treatment is meant to be lifelong and patients are advised not to discontinue thyroid replacement therapy when symptoms resolve. Patients are further advised to avoid calcium, iron supplements, grapefruit, soy, walnuts, and high fiber foods while taking these drugs orally, as they can impede absorption. Levothyroxine preparations are Yang-invigorating pharmaceuticals, and often result in Heat rising. This will be especially true if one already has signs of Heat or Liver Yang rising. Side effects include sensitivity to heat, sweating, hot flashes, fever, headache, insomnia, nervousness, anxiety, irritability, nausea, vomiting, appetite changes, and heart palpitations. Thyroid hormones may increase the metabolic clearance of glucocorticoids, and may cause adrenal crisis in those with adrenal insufficiency. Other medications, like insulin, may need to be adjusted when thyroid hormones are begun. It takes several weeks for L-thyroxine to take effect.

Liothyronine (L-T3): Cytomel. While T3 is the more active and Yang of the thyroid hormones with a greater therapeutic effect, it also has a short half-life, requires numerous doses daily, and is more unstable, causing serum levels to fluctuate. Cytomel is sometimes prescribed to those who don't respond well to levothyroxine. While most hypothyroid symptoms are resolved with T3 alone or in combination with T4, L-T3 has been associated with an increased risk of heart failure and stroke. While T3 can induce the same type of Heat symptoms that T4 does, it sometimes produces stronger and more erratic effects because of the increased Yang stimulation. Patients will often experience Heat signs that can harass the Heart.

Helping patients wean off thyroid medication requires patience commensurate with the length of time they have been taking them. If it has been less than a year, and there are no autoimmune factors to consider, tonify Kidney Yang, Spleen Qi, and Heart Blood as appropriate, and harmonize the Liver, while their prescribing physician monitors them to see if they can slowly wean off their meds. If they have been medicated for more than a year, expect it to take a while for their thyroid gland to "wake up." They may experience periods of lethargy and coldness, just like the symptoms of hypothyroidism, during which time they should cease cutting back on their medication as you continue to tonify Yang, Qi, and Blood, and clear any excesses that are present. If they have been medicated more than a few years, proceed with more caution; if it is over five years, it is less likely that they will be able to discontinue the medication entirely. It is not advisable to decrease thyroid medication during times of illness, pregnancy, or if the patient has plans to conceive in the near future.

Anti-thyroid agent

Methimazole (Tapazole, Narthex) is prescribed to treat hyperthyroid conditions like Graves' disease, or is given prior to radioactive iodine treatments or surgery of the thyroid gland. It acts directly on the thyroid gland to inhibit the incorporation of iodide into thyroglobulin, directly interfering with thyroid hormone production. Blocking the thyroid hormone reduces the symptoms of hyperthyroidism, but the range of possible side effects corresponds with the individual's underlying pattern and the extent of the hyperthyroidism. Because the thyroid hormone is associated with Yang and Wei Qi activity, side effects will diminish an array of Yang activity, commonly showing up with Qi stagnation and counterflow effects like stomach upset or pain, nausea, vomiting, headache, heartburn, dizziness, drowsiness and fatigue, numbness or tingling, rash, itching, hair loss, joint and muscle pain, chest tightness, and swellings.

The reproductive system and the hypothalamic-pituitary-ovarian axis

The reproductive system is a complex network of interaction between the organizing centers above and the output organs below. The hypothalamic-pituitary-ovarian (HPO) axis correlates with the flow between Ren Mai, Du Mai, and Chong Mai, all of which influence and are influenced by the Zang Fu. As Heaven pours down its pure Yang from the center of the Sea of Marrow, the life-giving Yin in the lower Dan Tien is activated. This powerful process steams the ongoing interaction of Fire and Water. The Triple Heater governs the steaming of Water as there is no vital Water without Fire to transform it, and no Fire of life without Water to fix it. San Jiao is a functional dynamic of how Yuan Qi is utilized, carrying in one network all of our Water-Fire interactions. The San Jiao network is in constant communication with the Pericardium, and thus its functions are largely impacted by our psychological and protective mechanisms. It is truly a "web which has no weaver."

The hypothalamus functions like a receiving station for antennae that perceive both outer and inner cues. The hypothalamus takes in enormous sensory data, processes it through our emotional response to our environment, and translates the input into pulsatile positive frequencies released in the form of gonadotropic releasing hormone (GnRH), and negative gonadotropic inhibitory hormone (GnIH) that will regulate the entire reproductive symphony of hormonal interaction. The pituitary gland then takes these impulses and interprets them into hormonal responses, releasing the pituitary-stimulating hormones FSH, LH, or PRL, along with inhibitory hormones to direct the downward precipitation of Tian Gui to Zi Gong—the palace of potential. Ovarian output is then steamed upward so the pituitary and hypothalamus assess what's going on down below, and can adjust their hormones accordingly.

Tian Gui is the Yin water which operates the reverse gynecological cycle of Early Heaven. This celestial dew was described as giving rise to the luxuriant grass on which the ancients poured the libations which they offered to the souls of the ancestors to keep the cycle of life going. In approximately two cycles of seven, Kidney Qi becomes exuberant, summoning the arrival of the heavenly elixir, Tian Gui. Through the Heart, the Mysterious Mother bestows the gift to bear life to the Uterus, the palace of potential, and the heavenly Essence of menses arrives as the woman synchs up with larger celestial rhythms. Ren Mai reaches upward to evaporate the fluids below, Yang Qi descends down Du Mai, and Chong Mai fills and empties along with the cycles of the moon.

The immortal Heng'e was known as goddess of the Moon, who presided over lunar cycles. Picture the moon rising from Ren 1 on the new moon until it reaches Du 20 during the full moon. This rise corresponds to the energetic ascent up the Chong Mai from the first day of the menstrual cycle until ovulation. Blood ascends to fill the Chong Mai, whose route of communication is said *to rise with vigor and circulate without fault to raise the heaviness of earth*. Chong Mai's great potential allows the Qi and Blood to circulate with precision, as the power of the Lower Jiao ascends to the ancestral Qi of the chest. Meanwhile, the Wei Qi descends one vertebral process per day, beginning with the hypothalamus at Du 17, Brain's Door, on Day Zero, as one menstrual cycle ends and the next begins. All hormones should be low this day, like the dark of the moon. On day 1 of bleeding, the Qi descends to the Wind Mansion at Du 16 to expel conflict from the marrow, and open and relax the four limbs as a new cycle begins. The Yin hormones from the ovary rise in response to FSH release from the pituitary gland as Blood begins to fill the Chong Mai. At ovulation Wei Qi descends behind the heart to Du 10 Soul's Tower, where it governs the inward movement below, determining which energies are allowed in. By day 21, the Wei Qi enters Ming Men where if life was sparked at ovulation, Destiny's Gate may open the route to Zi Gong if Heaven allows implantation to occur; otherwise, the Qi descends to the base of Du Mai where on the 28th day the Lungs release the old Blood and, as the moon rises, uterine blood again surges to recirculate and begin a new cycle. You can palpate the Ren Mai and Kidney channels up the front and Du Mai down the back for gummy areas of stuckness or flaccidity and, through needling, restore their proper flow.

Another goddess, Xi Wang Mu, the Queen Mother of the West, is said to occupy the nine mountain peaks in the head, where she directs the internal precipitation, filling the clouds through evaporation, and allowing them to shower down. Hers is the realm that bestows life and fertility, that honors the seven animal spirits that provide our earthly lessons, that governs the cycles of seven, bringing forth menarche and menopause, and of ongoing death and renewal. Therefore, she is the one who sits on the throne of the hypothalamus commanding the rhythms of the moon and the lunar cycles' reflection within the human female. As she doles out the celestial pulses, the pituitary gland releases FSH which stimulates one follicle which has been growing within the underworld of the ovary for many months, but has now been selected and primed to respond to its heavenly prompt to arise, grow, spew out estradiol, and release an egg. As long as we participate in honoring the cycles of life, our hormones flow in accordance. Where harmonizing reproductive hormones have cycled out of synch, this is mostly an inside job. In ancient times, the first remedy for menstrual cycle irregularities encouraged women to sleep under the moon for one full lunar cycle to realign with the Queen Mother's subtle internal dictates, spoken through the language of the changing moon.

When this internal celestial symphony is interrupted through the supplementation of hormones—any hormones—the natural cycles of Heaven are interrupted. Whether hormones are prescribed for fertility disorders or for the symptoms of menopause, it is as if we are telling Creation we know better. Instead of Heaven and Earth acting within and through the human being, humanity attempts to usurp the throne and vainly tries to govern earthly cycles, which is where most of our problems stem from to begin with.

Pituitary hormones of the reproductive cycle

Reproductive hormones rise and fall depending on the day of the menstrual cycle, and are impacted by climatic, environmental, and emotional factors. When blood work is drawn, "norms" are given, based on predictable, average 28-day cycles. Pituitary hormones are carried downstream by Lung Qi descending to help the Heart's warmth penetrate and vitalize the Yin hormones which, via the Kidneys, will grasp the Qi in the lower Jiao.

Follicle-stimulating hormone (FSH)

There is no "normal" FSH level. Values fluctuate based on age, day of menstrual cycle, certain medications, emotional shifts, and life stressors. FSH values taken on cycle day three, however, are considered a baseline prior to the rising energies on the conception meridian, and ideally should be below 10 mIU/ml in an ovulatory woman. FSH levels rise and fall, with the highest tide peaking around mid-cycle's full moon energies. As Chong Mai fills, the reproductive stream from the heavenly peaks in the head unleashes a hot spring whose current flows down from the pituitary gland with enough Yang to stimulate the primed follicle within the ovary to grow, produce estrogen, and release its egg. Levels are suppressed by the release of progesterone after ovulation.

FSH values are a measure of the Heart Yang that stimulates the Liver Blood and Kidney Yin to support the egg and estrogen production. We don't want too much of this Yang hormone, however. Elevated FSH levels are associated with either Yin-deficient Heat symptoms like hot flashes, night sweats, and irritability, or Liver Qi stagnation, when estrogen levels are often elevated as well.

High FSH levels indicate that the pituitary gland is working harder to stimulate the ovaries in order to get them to produce more estrogen. This may mean the ovaries (governed by the Kidneys) are deficient, in which case the Chi pulses will be weak or non-responsive, and not in communication with the Cun and Guan pulses. Elevations in FSH values are associated with Heat from Yin deficiency when estradiol levels are low as occurs in perimenopause and menopause. Zhi Bai di Huang Wan can help raise low estradiol and lower FSH in those with this pattern. Bear in mind that menses can pause due to climatic and emotional factors as well, so high FSH levels don't always indicate menopause. It generally means it takes more Yang to stimulate the unavailable Yin in the lower Jiao. This can be due to Yin deficiency where you will need to tonify Kidney and/or Liver Yin, or a Heart-Kidney imbalance, in which case Tian Wang Bu Xin Dang might be appropriate. When both estradiol and FSH are elevated, however, it correlates with Liver Qi stagnation—often with Heat, as the liver isn't able to metabolize either hormone, and they build up in the blood, losing their synchronization. Dan Zhi Xiao Yao San is often the best formula here. When the pattern is addressed, levels most often normalize until one approaches menopause. Also keep in mind there may be many other lifestyle and emotional factors that can be behind the Heart-Kidney imbalances.

Low FSH values are associated with Kidney Yang and Jing deficiency found in certain constitutional, hypothalamic, pituitary, or ovarian disorders, eating disorders, or when hormone therapy is given. Don't let terms like primary hypothalamic amenorrhea intimidate you. While they may be more challenging to treat, constitutional issues can still be addressed utilizing the Eight Extraordinary Vessels. Address the presenting pattern, utilize the Ren, Du, Chong, Wei, or Qiao Mai, and use one of the Essence tonifying formulas like You Gui Wan, Jin Gui Shen Qi Wan, or Si Wu Tang with Xian Mao, Yin Yang Huo, and the five seeds: Fu Pen Zi, Gou Qi Zi, Tu Si Zi, Che Qian Zi, and Wu Wei Zi.

During menopause, FSH values can rise to 30–240 mIU/ml. As the Ren and Chong Mai are no longer filling, the Heart and Kidneys cease their reproductive communication through Bao Mai, and the ovaries stop responding to FSH. I have worked with women whose premenopausal FSH levels were as high as 100 mIU/ml, who, when their patterns and underlying issues were resolved, returned to ovulatory cycles on their own and were able to conceive naturally. Note that those with extreme elevations of FSH will be unlikely to respond favorably to exogenous gonadotropin therapy.

Luteinizing hormone (LH)

As the follicle matures, Chong Mai ascends and estradiol levels peak, triggering the release of luteinizing hormone from the pituitary gland. LH is the hormone that is detected in ovulation predictor tests. Normal mid-cycle values should range from 6.17 to 17.2 mIU/mL. Luteinizing hormone is both warming and Qi moving, causing the egg to mature, and triggering its expulsion from the ovary approximately 36 hours after its surge. Ovulation is a process that is instigated by a full Heart and open Pericardium.

A process called luteinization describes how the follicle containing the egg transforms after the egg is released into a corpus luteum, or yellow body, associated with Earth energies, which will then begin to produce the warming hormone progesterone.

Because LH is released in response to rising ovarian hormones, we have to make sure Liver Blood and Kidney Yin are adequate and unobstructed to trigger the LH surge.

Low LH levels are seen in amenorrhea, anorexia, and other anovulatory disorders where LH isn't triggered because the Heart-Kidney axis is not communicating due to Blood or Yin deficiency. Jing is not being engaged, perhaps because of emotional tension. The Kidney pulses will feel very weak, and won't be communicating with the middle and upper Jiao energetics.

LH may become elevated when the Yang Qi is unable to trigger the egg's release due to Dampness or Phlegm, and/or the Liver Qi is stagnant. This scenario is often seen in polycystic ovary syndrome, where LH is released day after day, trying to get the ovary to release the egg, to no avail. Here the LH/FSH values will be high. While the entire cycle will need to be regulated, ovulatory strategies are to move the Qi, invigorate Blood, and resolve Dampness and Phlegm.

Because the release of the egg is ultimately governed by the Heart and Pericardium, after which the dynamic shifts to the Liver, ensure Liver Qi is harmonized, Liver Blood is adequate, and the Pericardium is unobstructed. Points like Lv 8, Lv 13, Lv 14, Pc 6, and Pc 8 might be appropriate to facilitate this release. Sometimes the most basic treatments like Yintang and the four gates may help synchronize the release of LH.

Reproductive hormones and folliculogenesis

The hundreds of thousands of primordial follicles contained within the ovaries remain unchanged until they are called out into circulation almost a year prior to their single chance at ovulation. Most of the follicles will not make it to the ovulatory finish line, but instead will be deselected along the way, and go into a state of atresia, never to be called out again. Protein synthesis, where egg quality is determined, occurs between 90 and 20 days prior to ovulation. This is a function of Yuan Qi, the Kidney-dominated push behind the ovarian response, and the Qi and Blood with which the developing follicle communicates. Egg quality cannot be improved on by reproductive procedures. Regardless of one's age, it is a process of harmonizing the inside with the outside.

Under normal circumstances, the ovaries will prime one chosen follicle from within, a function of Yuan Qi, to respond to small amounts of FSH. This dominant follicle, under the influence of Yang stimulation provided by FSH, will then respond to internal cues and grow to approximately 20 mm, during which time it is producing estrogen, which will trigger the release of LH from the pituitary gland to induce the release of the egg, and cause the follicle to be transformed into the progesterone-producing corpus luteum. The egg will travel through the corridor of the fallopian tube, where delicate cilia will sweep it toward the lumen of the uterus, and any sperm that have made it this far will then be given their chance to be selected to be capacitated and thereby contribute DNA to create a new life-giving combination.

The first "test tube babies" utilized in vitro fertilization to bypass mechanical issues such as blocked fallopian tubes. The naturally produced follicle was allowed to grow, its mature egg was then extracted, and placed in a Petri dish along with sperm to fertilize it. The resulting single embryo was then placed into the uterus where the expectant parents would wait to see if implantation took place. This allowed natural selection by the ovary, and allowed the egg to determine which sperm would be allowed in for fertilization. A few years later, a booming multi-billion dollar industry was born. As they do, drug companies figured out a way to capitalize on this novel interventional method. Reproductive clinics began to utilize hormones to inhibit the body's own regulatory hormones, suppress its own internal selection process, and manipulate the ovaries to overstimulate multiple follicles in order to manufacture the production of numerous eggs, which are then extracted via needle aspiration under ultrasound guidance. Natural selection went out of the window, as did the quality of eggs produced. But that's not all. Further interfering with natural selection, instead of placing egg and sperm together in the Petri dish and allowing fertilization to happen on its own, a new technological procedure called introcytoplamic sperm injection (ICSI) was employed where they whack off the sperms' tails, suck them into a needle, and inject them directly into the egg to force fertilization. While this process does produce babies, pregnancies conceived by this technology have much higher rates of complication and difficulty, including miscarriage, low birth weights, birth defects, and cardiovascular dysfunction in early life. It isn't the technology alone that is responsible for the dysfunction but the fact that if egg and sperm aren't capable of producing life on their own, there is greater likelihood for breakdown if fertilization is forced. Yet Heaven looks patiently on, allowing all of our attempts to outsmart nature.

Hormonal manipulation usually begins with the Dampening and Stagnating effects of oral contraceptives, followed by a GnRH agonst or antagonist to inhibit FSH and LH release and gonadal hormone output, the results of which can be very drying and depleting. Then very large doses of gonadotropins are administered via daily injection, which strongly invigorates the Yang to stimulate otherwise dormant follicles into circulation so their eggs can be extracted. Estrogen levels concurrently rise; often dramatically, which then causes the Blood to overfill and stresses the Liver. When it is necessary for a patient to take gonadotropins, you will often need to tonify Yin, Blood, and Jing, harmonize Liver Qi, and clear Heat and Dampness, while supporting their Kidneys. Yet an equally important job will be to help calm the Shen, as this can be quite an emotionally distraught process.

We will begin with pharmaceutical agents that impact the hypothalamic control of pituitary hormones, followed by pituitary hormones that act to manipulate gonadal output.

GnRH agonist and GnRH antagonists

GnRH agonist leuprolide (Lupron, Eligard) and *GnRH antagonists* cetrorelix (Cetrotide), ganirelix (Antagon, Fyremadel), elagolix (Orissa), relugolix (Orgovyx), degarelix (Firmagon), and abarelix (Plenaxis) prevent the release of estrogen or testosterone by holding back the pituitary release of FSH and LH. They are prescribed for certain conditions like precocious puberty, endometriosis, uterine fibroids, and prostate, testicular, breast, and ovarian cancers. They are also used to suppress the release of the body's own FSH and LH while gonadotropins are injected during in vitro fertilization cycles so the fertility drugs take over complete control of ovarian egg production without the interference of the body's own regulatory hormones. Lupron, as a stronger prototype, acts on the hypothalamus to block gonadal hormone release. Side effects are numerous and include loss of libido, impotence, hot flashes, night sweats, rashes, acne, general pain, headaches, dizziness, fatigue, weight loss, edema, loss of bone density, breast pain, vaginal dryness and swelling, breakthrough bleeding, decreased testicle size, and tremendous mood changes. Depression, emotional lability, and psychiatric events are not uncommon, especially in those with an underlying predisposition to mood disorders.

Pharmaceuticals that mimic GnRH effects act on the hypothalamus at the Ren Mai/Du Mai interface where they block Jing output and disrupt the Fire/Water balance. Severe Jing depletion will impact the production of Qi and

Blood. Because they deplete Kidney and Liver Yin, Yin-deficient Heat signs are common, as well as Dryness and Qi stagnation. Those with abundant Yin and Blood without Liver Qi stagnation will experience fewer side effects. While patients are taking Lupron, our treatment principles should include tonifying Kidney essence, Yin or Yang as needed, tonifying and moving Qi and Blood, clearing Heat, and calming the Shen. Practitioners often question whether prescribing herbs with phytoestrogenic effects (like Dang Gui and Xiang Fu) or testosterone-boosting effects (like Lu Rong and Ren Shen) will disrupt the drug's intended mode of action. (Bai Shao has phytoestrogenic effects but inhibits ovarian testosterone production.) At the doses we usually prescribe, effects are minimal; however, cautionary use is recommended. Select herbs with more Yin and Jing tonifying and astringent effects, like Nu Zhen Zi, Gou Qi Zi, Fu Pen Zi, and Wu Wei Zi, rather than those that directly tonify Qi and Blood, which tend to have more hormonally active effects.

Aromatase inhibitors

Clomiphene (Clomid, Serophene) and letrozole (Femara) are aromatase-inhibiting drugs with anti-estrogen effects, which were initially manufactured to treat estrogen receptor positive cancers. These molecules occupy the estrogen receptors, but instead of stimulating estrogen production, they inhibit estrogen's Yin- and Blood-enhancing effects on the cells. When they are used to stimulate ovulation, they are prescribed short term, tricking the body into producing more FSH to stimulate more follicles to produce increased numbers of eggs. The immediate effect is drying, potentially depleting Yin and inhibiting Blood generation in the endometrium. As the drugs are withdrawn, this is followed by a strong Yang effect, which stimulates Yin follicle production, and causes estrogen levels to rise, often far exceeding the norm, which dramatically causes Blood levels to rise, and often stagnates the Qi of the Liver and produces depressive Heat and/or Dampness. Falsely stimulating the movement of Essence can also result in Yin stagnation, which can develop into masses, and eventually reproductive cancers. Taking these drugs month after month can lead to cervical fluid too scant for sperm to swim through, and uterine linings too thin for implantation. Sometimes these drugs are just what a Yang-deficient patient needs short term, but they have the propensity to cause more long-term side effects, including endometrial cancer in patients who have issues other than Yang deficiency, which includes most of the modern Western patient population. Tonifying Yin and Blood while clearing Heat from FSH elevation and harmonizing the Liver can counteract the side effects of these drugs.

Anastrozole (Arimidex) is also an aromatase inhibitor that blocks estrogen's effects. Prescribed for estrogen positive breast cancers and pubertal gynecomastia, Arimidex is usually taken for about five years. As estrogen is a Yin- and Blood-enhancing hormone, aromatase inhibitors block Yin/Blood production. The Yin-depleting effects dry out the Damp environments in which cancers thrive, but can also consume the Yin and Blood and lead to Heat, producing side effects like hot flashes, blurred vision, light sensitivity and dizziness, heart rate variations, headache, nervousness, pounding in the ears, swelling of the lower legs, and bone pain.

Gonadotropins

Gonadotropins (FSH and LH) are hormones that are produced and released by the anterior pituitary gland to stimulate the ovaries and testes to produce sex hormones. Human chorionic gonadotropin (hCG) is another gonadotropin which is produced by the trophoblastic cells during pregnancy, and whose biologic actions are comparable to LH. These drugs are prescribed during fertility treatments to induce ovulation in women, and increase sperm counts in men. Most are injected subcutaneously, sometimes in doses as high as 450 mIU/day.

- Follicle-stimulating hormones (Gonal-f, Follistim, Puregon).
- Urofollitropins (Bravelle, Metrodin, Fertinex) are a form of purified FSH.
- Menotropins (Menopur, Repronex, Pergonal, Humegon) contain both FSH and LH.
- Lutropin alfa (Luveris, Pergoveris) is a recombinant luteinizing hormone.
- Human chorionic gonadotropin (hCG) (Pregnyl, Profasi, Novarel, Chorex, Pregnyl, Gonic, Chorigon, Choron-10).

Generally, when a person is prescribed gonadotropins for fertility treatments, their hormones have already been suppressed through GnRH agonists or antagonists. They also may have been on oral contraceptives to remove their own cyclical ovarian production of estrogen and progesterone. So they rarely begin the process in a harmonious state.

Gonadotropins have a Yang-stimulating effect, which may produce an overall feeling of warmth, with redness in the face, neck, arms, and upper chest. There will often be pain, swelling, and irritation at the injection sites, and as FSH stimulates follicular growth, estrogen levels rise, sometimes dramatically. Individuals may complain of back pain, breast tenderness, fatigue, irritability, frustration and anger, aches and pains, bloating, indigestion, pelvic and abdominal pain, shortness of breath, nausea, vomiting, or diarrhea. This is because the tremendous rise in both Yang and Yin hormones can result in countercurrent, Qi stagnation, Heat, and Dampness. As gonadotropin stimulation and ovarian hormones rise, a severe iatrogenic complication called ovarian hyper stimulation syndrome (OHSS) can develop where the ovaries exhibit an exaggerated reaction to the gonadotropins. Ovarian output explodes, and estradiol levels rise dramatically. The resulting increased capillary permeability causes fluids to leak out of the enlarging ovaries, making the abdomen swell, as patients become increasingly nauseous and uncomfortable. Intravascular hypovolemia is accompanied by severe edema and ascites; the swelling may impair diaphragmatic movement, potentially causing pulmonary dysfunction, respiratory distress, and hyper-coagulable states. Electrolyte imbalances and hypovolemia can lead to decreased renal perfusion and potentially acute renal failure. While the condition is most often self-limiting, the IVF cycle is usually cancelled. Patients can end up in intensive care, and may develop ruptured ovarian cysts and internal hemorrhages. If we are treating patients during the initial stages of OHSS, in addition to helping to alleviate their discomfort, we will be draining Dampness, working with the San Jiao, Kidney, Spleen, and Lung's control of fluids, and incorporating Water and Fire points.

Most of the effects of gonadotropins are due to the strong Yang stimulation leading to temporary overproduction of Yin, which then produces Dampness, in addition to Heat in the Blood. All hormones are metabolized by the liver, and Liver Qi stagnation is almost always a concomitant pattern. Because we are working with an unnatural procedure that forces abnormal ovarian stimulation, we can help by keeping the Qi and Blood moving, while directing the body's energies to the lower Jiao (e.g. e-Stim from UB 23 to UB 32, Sp 6, St 30, Ren 4). As the patients respond better to the medication, their reproductive endocrinologists can use lower doses for better ovarian response, although we don't want to try to mimic what the drugs are doing. Instead, we will want to clear Heat, while nourishing Yin. If your patients and their doctors allow herbal formulae, Kidney astringents, as listed above, as well as Tu Si Zi, Sang Ji Sheng, and Bai Shao, can also encourage more consistent follicular growth. Modify based on the pattern, incorporating Heat clearing and Qi harmonizing with appropriate tonification.

Overly stimulating the movement of hormones is a setup for hyper-proliferating Jing. We have known that stimulating hormones causes the body to lose Yin and release latency, putting mothers at higher risk for developing reproductive cancers later on. Yet it has only been within the last few years that studies are beginning to show the negative health consequences that gonadotropins have on the offspring of children conceived via IVF. Not only are complications during pregnancy and delivery more likely, these children have a much higher likelihood of developing hypertension during puberty.

Ovarian hormones

The endocrine system follows the Sheng cycle, as hormones have to harmonize with life first, while the gynecological cycle that belongs to the cosmic pre-heavenly flow operates in reverse. In the pre-heavenly realm, Blood, created by Earth, rises to be enlivened by Fire, which the Pericardium must cool and send to Wood's uprising power. The Liver must redirect the flow down to the Palace of Creation, governed by Water, where all new life arises. Together, the forward and reverse cycles operate like an infinity symbol; the entire symphony is directed by Metal, and Chong Mai brings it all together in the center.

Water, the source of life, ever seeks lower levels. The lower Jiao consists of Yin Water rising up from the depths like a spring, while Ming Men provides the Yang Fire to keep it moving. Because the spring water will pool without the activity of Fire to steam it upward, anything that interferes with this functional dynamic of the three burners can have a Dampening effect, which can settle in the basin of the lower Jiao. Dampening isn't only caused by substances; lack of appropriate physical or psychological movement can weaken the Spleen and dampen the spirits. Further, because the Gallbladder processes Ye fluids which can hold pathology latent, both hand and foot Shao Yang are involved in maintaining hormonal flow. The Gallbladder is also closely related with the Dai, Yang Wei, and Yang Qiao Mai. Thus, psychological and life issues that we have not dealt with often can cause these Extraordinary Meridians to accumulate pathology and impact the smooth flow of hormones. Many perimenopausal hormonal issues that occur during the vulnerable cycles of seven are resolved by facing fears and regrets, and making new decisions as one enters into new phases of life.

The Yang hormones from the pituitary gland trigger the more Yin hormones from the ovary. In reproductive and adrenal hormonal circuitry, cholesterol makes up the fatty substance Ye, the precursor of glucocorticoids, mineralocorticoids, androgens, and estrogens. When shunted down the reproductive pathway, cholesterol is transformed into pregnenolone, which is made into progesterone by the corpus luteum. Pregnenolone also transforms into 17-OH pregnenolone, which then becomes DHEA, which is converted to androstenedione and gives rise to testosterone (in a Yang environment), or estrone, and eventually the active hormone estradiol E2 in a Yin environment.

The conversion from androstenedione to estrone occurs via an enzyme in fat tissue called aromatase. In the absence of Yin aromatase, 17-beta hydroxysteroid dehydrogenase converts androstenedione to the more Yang testosterone. This is a very important point for those who supplement with the steroid precursor DHEA. In a Yang-deficient environment, DHEA can help move toward estradiol production; however, in a Yang-excess, Yin-deficient milieu, DHEA can be shunted toward the testosterone pathway instead of estradiol. This can manifest with irritability, aggression, acne, loss of head hair, development of facial hair, and pubic hair that extends up toward the navel. DHEA is warming and should not be administered to a Yin-deficient patient with signs of Heat or Stagnation; until the excess is cleared, it will only worsen these presentations.

Pregnenolone is converted directly to progesterone, but has to go through more conversion steps to reach estrogen or testosterone. It has more of a Jing tonifying effect, and is more effective for those with Heat signs.

Estrogen and progesterone are the active hormones that plug into cellular receptors as they perform essential functions within the cell.

Estradiol (E2)

The human ovary produces three types of estrogen: Estrone E1, a precursor of estradiol that becomes dominant during menopause; estradiol E2, the strongest and most active reproductive hormone; and estriol E3, the milder form which is produced in higher amounts during pregnancy. We will be concerned with the active hormone estradiol E2.

Estradiol is the major hormone in the body that has functional properties of both Yin and Blood. Primarily produced by the ovary, estradiol rises from 30 pmol/mL (taken on day three) to up to 400 pmol/mL mid-cycle. Estrogen causes our primary and secondary sexual characteristics, holds on to moisture, and affects the urinary tract, heart, blood vessels, breasts, bones, skin, hair, mucous membranes, and pelvic muscles. All of these effects belong to Kidney Yin, Liver Yin, Liver Blood, and Heart Blood.

Estrogen dominates the Yin or follicular phase of the menstrual cycle—after menses until ovulation. The dominant follicle produces estradiol, which rises daily until the pituitary gland perceives it has reached its optimum level and initiates signals to mature the egg and induce ovulation; thereafter estradiol levels plateau and fall toward the end of the cycle. Rising estradiol also makes the endometrium proliferate and thicken; it produces and thins cervical mucus; and lifts, opens, and softens the cervical opening as ovulation approaches to allow sperm to enter. It then triggers the release of LH so the egg can be discharged into this lush environment that sperm live for.

Low estradiol levels indicate deficient Kidney Yin, Liver Yin, Liver Blood, or Heart Blood. Yin-deficient Heat signs like hot flashes and night sweats are often present, and Blood stasis often accompanies Blood deficiency. Cervical fluid may be lacking, and sexual desire may be low. The endometrium tends to be thin and menses more scant. When the presenting pattern includes Yin-deficient Heat, the follicular phase is usually short, not giving the egg adequate time to mature. Treatment includes tonifying Yin and Blood, clearing Heat, and moving the Blood. Zhi Bai di Huang Wan, Liu Wei di Huang

Wan, Si Wu Tang, Gui Pi Tang, Zuo Gui Wan, and Da Bu Yin Wan are good Yin and Blood tonifying formulas. Choose from points such as: Sp 6, Sp 4, Ki 3, Zi Gong Xue, St 30, UB 23, UB 32, UB 52, and Sp 10.

Estrogen makes things grow. If excess estrogen builds up in the consolidating environment of the uterus, it can gather into accumulations like fibroids, endometriosis, and estrogen-sensitive tumors. Accumulation of Yin estrogen produces a Damp environment, and because the liver metabolizes hormones, high estradiol levels are also associated with Liver Qi stagnation, often with Heat. Many times, women with elevated estradiol levels will experience bloating, breast tenderness and irritability around ovulation, and more severe pre-menstrual symptoms, indicating that estrogen is accumulating.

Estrogen dominance is a condition where estradiol levels build up—not only from ovarian production, but also through pharmaceutical estrogens, and dietary ingestion of estrogenic compounds which also leak into our water supplies. Our environment contains many forms of estrogen disrupters—glyphosate, phthalates, polychlorinated biphenyls (PCBs), dioxins, and so on, used in pesticides, industrial solvents, and plastics. Xenoestrogens are foreign chemicals that are molecularly similar to estrogens, and bind strongly to the estrogen receptor sites to wreak potentially hazard consequences. Phytoestrogens, contained in foods like soy and herbs like Dang Gui and Xiang Fu, however, can preferentially displace the xenoestrogens. Fibroids, endometriosis, and many reproductive cancers are worsened by estrogen dominance. Usually the Blood becomes stagnant from the Liver's inability to metabolize excess estrogen. In the case of endometriosis, we know the Bao Mai, the carrier of life's potential, becomes inflamed. Anti-endometrial antibodies may be present, indicating that Wei Qi is now reacting against the autointoxication caused by estrogen disruption.

The patterns behind fibroids and endometriosis include Qi stagnation, Dampness, Phlegm, Toxic Heat, and/or Blood stasis, often with an underlying vacuous condition. Check the pulse proximal to the Left Chi for the quality. In most cases of estrogen dominance, it does not help the underlying cause to add progesterone to balance out the excess. The Liver needs to be decongested: Xiao Chai Hu Tang, Xiao Yao San, Dan Zhi Xiao Yao San, Lv 2, Lv 3, Lv 14. Dandelion greens and leafy green vegetables help the Liver metabolize excess, and cruciferous vegetables contain diindolylmethane (DIM), which improves the enzyme activity of estrogen metabolism. Regulating the colon is also extremely important to rid the body of excess estrogen levels that the Liver has processed.

Progesterone (P4)

After the egg is released, the dominant follicle transforms into a corpus luteum, which starts to manufacture progesterone during the luteal phase. In a normal menstrual cycle, blood progesterone levels should remain low until after ovulation. Blood tests are usually taken on day 21 of the menstrual cycle (assuming ovulation happened on day 14) and then progesterone should range from 10 to 20 ng/mL. P4 has more of a warming effect than estrogen, and raises the body temperature almost half of a Fahrenheit degree. It is like the Yang within Yin. If an embryo implants in the uterine lining, it sends out beta hCG, which triggers the corpus luteum to release more progesterone, raising the body temperature to support the Yang needs of the developing pregnancy. Progesterone can cause bloating, breast tenderness, and food cravings. Here Kidney Yang is helping the Spleen to bank the Blood; excess levels can cause excess holding, resulting in Damp retention and swelling. Progesterone influences the endometrium to reveal a secretory pattern wherein the glands become full, the arteries engorge, and the connective tissue swells in preparation for implantation.

Low progesterone levels are most often due to Kidney Yang and Spleen Qi deficiency; but can also be the result of a follicle that didn't grow adequately during the follicular phase due to Yin and Blood deficiency. Herbs with a high sticky content like Shan Yao, Da Zao, E Jiao, and Yi Tang can help, and yams are known to raise progesterone levels. Bu Zhong Yi Qi Tang can help with sunken Spleen Qi, as well as Yang tonics like Du Zhong, Xu Duan, and Zi He Che. Topical progesterone cream can raise progesterone levels, but progesterone supplementation isn't known to help with implantation if the follicle was unable to produce a healthy corpus luteum. Ki 2, Ki 7, Sp 3, Sp 8, Ren 6, St 36, and Du 20 can help tonify Yang and lift the Qi.

High progesterone levels are not common unless one is pregnant or has been supplementing progesterone. Then it acts like physiologic Damp Heat. Unlike estrogen, which lingers in the blood, progesterone has a very short half-life. If overly supplemented, progesterone can build up in the fatty tissues over time, inhibiting the proper drop in progesterone necessary to bring on the period, disrupting the menstrual cycle.

Androgens

Androgens are present in both males and females, but are responsible for more of the hormone-associated male traits. Androstenedione is a weak androgenic steroid produced mostly by the testes, but also the ovary and adrenal gland. It is an androgenic precursor to both testosterone and estrone.

Testosterone

Normal levels are considered to be normal when they call between 300 and 1000 ng/dL. Produced mainly by the testicles, testosterone is the primary male sex hormone responsible for sperm production, masculinization, muscle mass, and sex drive. While hormones are generally considered more Yin, testosterone has a stronger Yang, Heating effect. Testosterone levels drop as men age; they can also rise and fall when a man is in an environment that does or doesn't allow him to exert his dominant male characteristics. It isn't unusual for a man who has lost his job or whose partner has a more dominant role in the relationship to have lowered testosterone. Increasing activities like competitive sports can help his vital Qi return, often along with testosterone levels. Phytoestrogens found in soy and dairy products, alcohol, and a diet high in breads, pastries, and desserts can lower testosterone levels as well. Testosterone can be elevated with exposure to sunlight, exercise, competitive games, having sex, D-aspartic acid, DHEA, adaptogens like Ren Shen and Ashwagandha, and Yang tonifying herbs like Lu Rong.

When testosterone is low, men often experience symptoms like erectile dysfunction, low libido, and low sperm counts, and they may feel as if they are lacking vitality and have poor energy levels. They may lose facial and body hair, experience decrease in lean muscle mass and an increase in body fat, have difficulty concentrating, and become depressed.

Testosterone replacement therapy isn't normally given orally, as there can be negative effects on the liver. It can be delivered by transdermal skin patches (Androderm), gels (AndroGel, Testim, Axiron, Fortesta, Natesto), mouth patches (Striant), injections, and implants. While symptoms of low testosterone often improve with supplementation, there are dangers in taking testosterone, such as increased risk of heart attacks and strokes, aggressive behavior, worsening of benign prostatic hypertrophy and prostate cancer, sleep apnea, blood clots, and congestive heart failure. These side effects are primarily due to rising Heat and Damp Heat.

Dihydrotestosterone (DHT) is a metabolite of testosterone produced by the testes and skin. It binds strongly to androgen receptors on the cell, with a greater Yang effect than testosterone. DHT promotes sebaceous gland activity, growth of facial and pubic hair, as well as male pattern baldness and potentially dangerous prostate growth. DHT blockers like finasteride, used to prevent hair loss, can also cause erectile dysfunction because of the loss of Yang stimulation. Saw Palmetto and turmeric are healthy alternatives for DHT elevations.

Ovarian hormonal therapy

Because of the negative feedback loop that maintains cyclical hormonal homeostasis, biomedical hormonal management only temporarily manages specific desired outcomes; but they shouldn't be considered curative nor safe. Hormonal manipulation will always result in the potential for side effects, some quite severe, although often overlooked.

Hormonal contraceptives

Different types of oral contraceptives include combined estrogen and progesterone, either in monophonic pills that provide a steady dose of hormones throughout the cycle, with graduated amounts of estrogen and progesterone for 21 days and placebo pills for seven days, or continuous use where active hormones are taken for a year at a time, which stops all menstrual bleeding. There is also the extended use pill, where one takes active hormones for three months, followed by a week off when bleeding occurs, as well as progesterone-only pills and implantable devices. They are all intended to emit progesterone and/or estrogen into the bloodstream to prevent pregnancy through various means. The combined contraceptives are too numerous to list, as they would take up this entire chapter. Each may be composed of a blend of synthetic estrogen, such as ethinyl estradiol, and progestins like norethindrone; they may exclusively contain progestin such as medroxyprogesterone (Provera), or implantable progestin release like etono-gestrel. They may come in the form of intrauterine devices (IUDs) like Mirena, plastic T-shaped devices that are placed in the uterus to emit progestins into the bloodstream. There are also progestin pills taken after unprotected sex, like levonorgestrel emergency contraceptives (Morning After). When we understand what exogenous estrogens and progestins do in the body, we can understand them all.

Estrogen has Yin- and Blood-promoting effects. Application of synthetic estrogen administration inhibits follicular development by its effect on the anterior pituitary gland, which in response to estrogen decreases FSH secretion. In excess, the moistening effects of estrogen have Stagnating and Dampening properties, especially in the absence of Yang to move the excess Yin. Progesterone is also Yin, but with more Yang effects. External progesterone administration inhibits follicular development and ovulation via negative feedback to the hypothalamus, disrupting the pulse frequency of GnRH, which reduces FSH and LH. Progestins also make the cervical mucus inhospitable to sperm penetration as well as altering endometrial thickness, a process which inhibits implantation when it's out of sync with natural menstrual cycling. Some progestins have antiandrogenic properties that can reduce the hirsutism and acne associated with polycystic ovary syndrome. Progesterone encourages the growth of new tissues, as during the luteal phase it warms and endows the endometrium with new circulation and the ability to secrete substances which will feed an implanting embryo. This Yang Qi in the depth of Yin allows the Qi to hold, although long-term progesterone administration has Dampening and congestive qualities like impairing glucose metabolism, stagnating the Qi, and potentially depleting Kidney Qi.

The mechanisms of oral contraceptives that inhibit ovulation and reduce menstrual flow give rise to side effects such as nausea, vomiting, water retention, weight gain, breast tenderness, thromboembolic episodes, hypertension, strokes, the potential for myocardial infarctions, and breast and endometrial cancers. All hormonal contraceptives have the tendency to cause Dampness, Qi stagnation, and Blood stasis. Continuous use contraceptives stagnate the

Qi, Blood, and body fluids more than the monthly pills, which at least allow the hormonally rich blood to be released each month.

Synthetic estrogenic compounds in our food supply and drinking water already overburden our systems with their toxic and potentially carcinogenic effects. We should be wary of the effects of administering more hormones into our system. Contraceptive hormonal therapy provides exogenous Ye supplementation that disrupts the natural internal hormonal processing, which can, based on the individual's underlying pattern, lead to Dampness, Liver Qi stagnation, Heat, and/or Blood stasis. Those with fewer patterns of imbalance will tend to have fewer side effects; however, all hormonal supplementation can lead to congested Qi and Blood.

Menopause

As a woman approaches the end of her reproductive years, she moves from Jing dominance toward Shen dominance. Any unmet psychological issues, or lifestyle that goes against the destiny of one's true nature, will produce conflicts in the Qi. Many, if not most, menopausal symptoms are caused by internal conflicts that stagnate the Qi, causing Heat to develop as the Qi shifts from the Ministerial Fire to the Sovereign Fire in the chest.

During the perimenopausal transition, which may begin in the late thirties and last until menopause (the average age of menopause is now 52 rather than 49, largely due to hormonal excesses), changes occur not only in the ovaries, but in the hypothalamus and pituitary gland. Changes occur in the pulsatile release of GnRH and configurations of FSH. Menstrual cycle patterns often become erratic, as does estradiol output. Eventually, FSH and LH stop communicating with the ovaries, and menses ceases. Estradiol levels drop dramatically because they are meant to; eventually estrone exceeds estradiol levels. The Liver also processes these hormones differently now. When the Liver is congested, instead of metabolizing to 2-hydroxyestrone, both estradiol and estrone can be converted to excess 16-alpha hydroxyestrone, a more toxic metabolite which promotes estrogen-dependent cancers. Emotional resistance to menopause stagnates the Liver; and the time it takes to transition from perimenopause into the threshold of menopause is dependent on the state of the Liver.

When the retiring ovaries cease Yin production and estrogen decreases, the nervous system can experience a withdrawal-type effect, and a mutual transference in Kidney Yang causes the adrenal gland to release surges of norepinephrine. Yang escapes from the lower Jiao and floats upwards, causing Heat signs like hot flashes, night sweats, insomnia, and anxiety. As the Ming Men Fire is displaced, exuberant Liver Yang rises along with it, sometimes resulting in hypertension. As Dampness compensates for Yin-deficient Heat, cortisol levels may rise. Thyroid metabolism may become dysregulated, and weight increases. Cholesterol production increases to try to produce more of the raw material to manufacture steroids. As Heat increases, the body tries to neutralize the acidic environment by extracting calcium from the bones, a process which may lead to osteopenia.

Root Kidney Yang and support the adrenal glands: Du 4, Ren 4, UB 22, UB 23, UB 52. Formulae like Er Xian Tang are given for this purpose. Modify with Yin tonics; clear Liver Heat, resolve Damp accumulation, and calm the Shen. Help open the Heart and Pericardium. Working with the Eight Extraordinary Vessels that form the energy vortex at the center of the body can help support someone who is being welcomed into her wisdom years.

Menopause is not a disease, and hormones are not the solution. The body wants to stop producing and processing estrogen and progesterone; even bioidentical hormones can Dampen and stagnate the Qi, which can exacerbate all kinds of negative symptoms, including depression. The prevailing conventional medical narrative tells us we need to take estrogen for bone strength and cardiovascular health. Since we know that nature didn't err, however, we can see that as Yin declines, we are called to shift any residual excess Yang movements that our heart and bones can no longer withstand. The transformative Fire of the menopausal transition is meant to burn off any unhealthy patterns that were not addressed earlier in life so we can move past residual egoic drives for emotional gratification and relax into a more Heart-centered life. This is the time to face the dark heavy places so they can be left behind, although they may not remain asymptomatic. Mood changes are common, including depression, anxiety, and irritability. Rarely do these types of changes leave the psyche untouched. Perimenopause is an opportunity to face ourselves and courageously step into the journey destined by our souls. It might be hard work to follow Chong Mai's blueprint to raise the heaviness of Earth as the power of the lower Jiao ascends to the ancestral Qi in the Chest. If we follow this great inner power, however, Shen are redeemed from Jing, and we become lighter in step and demeanor as pre- and post-heaven meet to rectify the HPO axis, the thyroid, and adrenal glands. Rooted in spirit, we ascend from our own depths and the proper movement of life is given from within rather than without.

Menopausal hormone replacement therapy

Menopausal hormonal replacement therapy is prescribed for women in their perimenopausal or post-menopausal years who complain of symptoms such as hot flashes, night sweats, vaginal dryness, loss of interest in sex, insomnia, anxiety, irritability, and depression. HRT preparations include:

- Estradiol (Estrace, Delestrogen, Divigel, Elestrin, Estradot, Estrasorb, Estrogel, Evamist, Femtrace)
- Estropipate (Ogen, Ortho-Est)
- Conjugated estrogens (Premarin)
- Esterified estrogens (Menest)
- Estradiol injections (Depo-Estradiol)
- Vaginal creams (Estrace Vaginal, Estring, Vagifem, Yuvafem)
- Vaginal ring (Estring, Femring)
- Patches (Alors, Climara, Minivelle, Estraderm, Vivelle-dot, Menostar)
- Spray (Evamist)

Estrogen and progestin hormone therapy: Activella contains estradiol and norethindrone acetate. Angeliq is composed of estradiol and drospirenone. Prempro and premphase contain conjugated estrogens and medroxyproges-terone acetate.

We have described the mechanism of estrogens and progestins above. All estrogen-containing preparations can cause fluid retention, swelling, breast pain, lumps or breast cancers, vaginal itching, discharge or bleeding, endo-metrial cancer, gallstones, blood clots, strokes, and heart attacks. Side effects also include Gl upset, stomach pain, bloating, nausea, diarrhea, weight gain, headache, dizziness, lightheadedness, mood changes, sleep changes, vaginal itching, bleeding, spotting, breast pain or tenderness, swelling, and bloating. Any time we artificially supplement Yin with hormone replacement therapy, we can also upset the Yang thyroid hormones.

Of course, we can utilize our skills addressing the side effects caused by the Dampening, Stagnating, and Blood clotting effects of HRT, and then helping them through the carcinogenic or cardiovascular damage caused by them. Or we can tonify the Kidney Yin and Yang, Qi, and Blood, harmonize the Qi, move the Blood, calm the Shen, and support our patients as they remain conscious of what their symptoms represent. It can be a powerful part of the healing profession to support someone as they learn to recognize and participate with the wisdom of their bodies. Without hormones muting the experience, they can witness their Qi rising and express unacknowledged anger; they can see how the descending nature of fear has been holding them back from living fully; and they can begin to embrace the opportunity to rid the toxic emotional stagnation that may have been festering for years.

Bone loss, osteopenia, and osteoporosis treatment

Post-menopausal bone loss coincides with the reduction in estrogen levels. That does not necessarily mean that low estrogen levels *cause* bone loss. Many factors contribute to this condition, which begins at around age 35 when the body's production of new bone by osteoblasts slows down, but the reabsorption of old bone by osteoclasts does not, resulting in a condition called osteopenia, a natural process of aging. While age-related hormonal changes in women contribute, so do lack of weight-bearing exercises, poor diet, caffeine, smoking, drinking alcohol, and certain medications like prednisone. When the condition progresses to osteoporosis, back pain, stooped posture, and loss of height may indicate that the bones are more brittle and prone to fracturing. Bone loss is diagnosed with dual-energy x-ray absorptiometry, which provides a negative score indicating the amount of bone loss and whether osteopenia has progressed to osteoporosis.

The mechanism of rapid bone loss is largely due to Heat, often from underlying Kidney Yin deficiency, although any type of Heat in the Blood or Toxic Heat can be responsible. Calcium is then leached from the bone to neutralize the inflammation. Weakening bones indicates Kidney deficiency, and

Kidney tonics can help, as can herbal formulae with Long Gu and Mu Li, such as Chai Hu Jia Long Gu Mu Li Tang, depending on the pattern. UB 11, the Hui meeting point of bone, and GB 39, the meeting point of marrow, should be used along with treating whatever patterns of imbalance are present. Exercise, mineral-rich diets, and reducing inflammatory substances including alcohol and smoking will help, as well as supplementing with vitamin D, calcium, magnesium, and boron, which helps build back the bone. Weight-bearing exercises also encourage new bone formation. Estrogen and progestin medications used to be prescribed to treat osteoporosis, but because of the increased risk of blood clots and breast and endometrial cancer, they are usually reserved for those who cannot take other osteoporosis drugs.

Osteoporosis medication

Raloxifene (Evista) is an estrogen receptor modulator prescribed to address osteoporosis in post-menopausal women. Evista, which is not a hormone, binds to estrogen receptors where it alters the expression of genes that maintain bone density. It also reduces the risk of invasive breast cancer in those at risk, although it is not a cancer drug. Evista interferes with the movement of Qi and Blood, and its stagnating effect increases the risk of blood clots. Other side effects include chest pain, difficulty breathing, leg cramps, joint pain, swelling, nausea and flu-like symptoms, increased risk of infection, hot flashes, sweating, headaches, and increased urge to urinate.

Other pharmaceuticals which are offered for the pharmacological management of osteoporosis include biphosphonates like alendronate (Fosamax), which is a weekly pill, risedronate (Actonel), a weekly or monthly pill, ibandronate (Bonita), a monthly pill or quarterly intravenous infusion, or zoledronic acid (Reclast), an annual intravenous infusion. These drugs reduce the rate at which calcium is lost from the bones. Biphosphonates are not absorbed well, and often produce stomach pain, nausea, acid reflux, diarrhea, bloating, headaches, and inflammation. They can also cause osteonecrosis of the jaw and breaks in the femur. Keeping calcium in the bone may prevent bone deterioration, but we have to ask how it affects the Heat that the calcium is attempting to neutralize. By inhibiting the settling effect minerals have in the blood, underlying Heat and inflammation can worsen. These drugs also stagnate the Qi, especially in the upper GI tract, causing severe counterflow, and may even cause esophageal cancer.

Denosumab (Prolia, Xgeva) is a monoclonal antibody which inhibits osteoclast formation to reduce the breakdown of bones. It is administered subcutaneously every six months and can cause weight gain, eczema, cellulitis, and osteonecrosis of the jaw. Its therapeutic effects do not continue after treatment is halted, and discontinuing the medication may cause a rebound effect resulting in bone fractures. Inhibiting osteoclast bone resorption blocks Heat but does not clear it, which may cause the Heat to translocate to other sites. Bone-building drugs include teriparatide (Forteo), abaloparatide (Tymlos), injected daily, and romosozumab (Evenity), injected monthly for 12 months. Teriparatide and abaloparatide may potentially increase the likelihood of developing bone cancer. Bone-building drugs are taken for a year or two, and then stopped, after which their effects will quickly diminish, so patients are often switched to a biphosphonate thereafter. Low calcium levels in the blood can induce an array of side effects, including joint pain, muscle spasms, neck pain, swelling of the hands and feet, weakness, headaches, insomnia, as well as numbness and itching in the arms, hands, legs, and feet. More severe side effects include increased risk of strokes and heart attacks. Kidney-nourishing tonics, on the other hand, can help increase bone mineral density without negative side effects.

CHAPTER 10

Cancer and Chemotherapeutic Agents

Chinese medicine doesn't treat cancer; it doesn't even have a word to define the concept of cancer. We, of course, treat individuals who may have received Western diagnoses of cancer, and through various healing modalities like Chinese medicine, they often overcome their malady with or without conventional allopathic treatments. Cancer isn't actually a thing, like a noun; it's more of a process, like a verb, that describes the dysfunctional proliferation of cells. This process goes on in everyone, but the immune system usually takes care of the aberrant cells without our knowledge.

Tumorous growths, however, actually are substantial things and Chapter 81 of the *Ling Shu* is devoted to swellings and their treatment. The gist is to treat the pattern, but leave the swellings alone. If you cut into them, we are warned, you can cause death. Even Hippocrates said to leave tumorous growths alone, to allow the body to heal itself. So if we don't cut them, what strategies are we left with? To ascertain and address the root, offering natural remedies while the cure takes place. While Hippocrates is claimed as the father of Western medicine, his rebellious son changed all of this. Cutting out tumors is now most often the first approach, followed by cytotoxic drugs and irradiation. This is one of the most horrific treatments a human being can undergo, but not the only route available. The point I hope to make is that there are other valid approaches, Chinese medicine being one of them, and all patients should be encouraged to make informed decisions for themselves.

How people receive and respond to a cancer diagnosis can influence the choices they make or even determine the outcome. From a state of resistance and fear, the Qi will be constricted, leading to rash decisions, reducing one's ability to see the whole and act from the highest good. Taoist practices are always encouraging non-resistance, which does not mean we just roll over and take it. Non-resistance is a powerful stance which simply doesn't fight what is. If an individual is supported to remain in a state of acceptance, strength, and wisdom, they may be able to pause and redirect their vision. Perhaps they may become aware of any underlying conditions that may have created the internal environment that has predisposed them to manifesting tumors or invasive Fire toxins, as the case may be, in the first place. I'm not suggesting that all of our Qi and Blood should be directed toward uncovering concealed psychogenic factors. In the case of childhood cancers, for instance, we would be wasting our time delving into personal causation. But as you well know, the Chinese medical view goes much deeper than the appearance of things. All recipients of cancer are, to some extent, products of their ancestry, conditioning, environment, and lifestyle. But one's state of mind is a much larger player than we usually allow. So perhaps we can begin to serve our patients best by helping them advocate for themselves, navigate their own treatment options, and invest their Heart-Minds to influence the outcome in a positive way.

The fear-based approaches which dominate the conventional oncological methods seek for the most effective means of destroying the tissues and killing the manifestation, regardless of the cost. And the cost is great, whether to the body, mind, or pocketbook. Cancer drugs generate extremely high revenues—hundreds of billions of dollars annually, and rising, driven by the fear of death. Yet cancer rates continue to rise, and despite the money allocated for research, medicine is no closer to curing it, but just perpetuating ongoing treatment. We seem to be stuck in a loop that we don't know how to get out of, which is fueled by the fact that our greatest health fear is of developing and dying from cancer.

Many patients are traumatized by the cancer diagnosis itself, which causes shock and fear, depleting the Kidneys and shutting down the source of the body's immunity. This level of resistance is capable of creating as much pathology as the disease itself. Just as cancer is the result of loss of internal regulatory control, the patients may lose regulatory control of their own care. Decisions based on fear do not engage the capacity for the patients to fully advocate for themselves in calm, rational, and proactive ways. Someone who is fearful is more inclined to do whatever therapy is suggested, for fear if they don't, the cancer will win (and kill them) and they will lose (and be killed). Even if they are inclined to address their diagnosis with a more natural approach, their families may become reactive, steering the patient to adhere to "real" medicine. Any movement outside conventional recommendations may add guilt to the underlying fear, further stagnating the Qi. As they move further into the system, legal documents must be signed, often when patients are at their most fearful, that lock in extreme measures to keep them alive and out of pain for as long as possible, regardless of the quality of life. This "fight for life" puts them in the process of already dying, at least in their minds. It can be a real setup to blindly accept conventional cytotoxic approaches, and perhaps regret the decisions afterwards.

There are endless natural remedies for cancer, though not FDA approved. A quick internet search can lead down a rabbit hole of supplements and herbs, along with admonitions like *studies haven't shown anti-cancer activity, ask your doctor first, these may interfere with the effectiveness of chemotherapy...* This usually causes so much confusion and the patient defaults to accepting that their doctor knows best. Yet there is very little allopathic medical education devoted to diet, health, and wellness, so we're mostly on our own in this territory.

We have all heard of natural diets and nutritional supplements that are effective against cancer. The "anti-cancer diet" attempts to remove all preservatives, refined carbohydrates, genetically modified grains, sugars, and unhealthy fats from the diet. This shouldn't be just an anti-cancer diet, but the ongoing dietary plan we all abide by. While it keeps many toxic food substances out of the body, it doesn't "fight" cancer. Other foodstuffs that haven't been patented, artificially modified, and marketed by pharmaceutical companies offer promise, but nobody is interested in funding research that doesn't benefit the industry. Apple seeds, for example, contain vitamin B17, or amygdalin, a nitrioside that occurs naturally in various edible plants, seeds, berries, and nuts. In these plants, each amygdalin molecule wraps up one hydrogen cyanide unit within benzaldehyde and glucose. But our bodies don't carry the enzyme to unbind the cyanide, unless we happen to harbor cells which are replicating out of control. Yes, as nature would have it, only cancer cells contain the beta-glucosidase enzyme that can unwrap and release the cyanide into circulation, targeting the cancer cells.

Laetrile (Dorr & Paxinos, 1978; Moss, 1996; Rauws, Olling, & Timmerman, 1982), a synthetic form of amygdalin, whose active ingredient was hydrogen cyanide, was first used as a cancer treatment in Russia in the mid-1800s, and in the US in the 1920s. In the 1970s, mainstream oncology and anti-cancer pharmacological approaches rejected the validity of the research which was the basis of Laetrile treatments, stating it showed little "anti-cancer activity." In 1980, the FDA declared its sale to be against federal law, and while it is illegal to market and sell amygdalin in the United States and Europe, it isn't against the law to eat apple seeds. Apples have many other anti-cancer properties as well. I'm pretty sure the Tao did not err in failing to alert horses, squirrels, and deer of the poisonous effects of apple seeds so they could eat around the core, like their whacky human cousins have trained themselves to do.

In an article published in *Biomolecules* in 2019 (Rosse de Souza *et al.*, 2019), bioactive compounds found in Amazonian fruits murici and tapereba were reported to have potent cytotoxic effects on ovarian cancer cells. Another study, in *Integrative Cancer Therapies* (Ruochen Dong, Ping Chen, & Qi Chen, 2018), reported the effects of pao pereira, an extract from a South American tree bark, which was found to inhibit proliferation of pancreatic cancer cells. Injections of mistletoe extract are one of the most widely prescribed natural treatments for cancer in Europe. These therapies have been effective at stalling the growth and spread of cancer cells, but since clinical trials in the US are lacking, the FDA has not approved their use in the treatment of cancer. If pharmaceutical companies can't synthesize the remedy, it is usually scrapped and its healing benefits are hidden from public view. If the cure is really promising, patents will be taken out by those who already monopolize the pharmaceutical industry to prevent others from developing these remedies further.

This happened to Zach Bush, MD, who, when his promising cancer treatment patent was bought out from under him, was sent in a new direction entirely. In an interview published in *Salon Magazine*, Bush said, "I went from that world of chemotherapy and drug concepts and drug development to the sudden realization that there had never been a cancer caused by a lack of chemotherapy… And so, no matter how good I got at making chemotherapy, I was always going to be missing the point, missing the root cause of the situation" (Karlis, 2019). Bush opened a nutrition center in rural Virginia, which led him to discover the carcinogenic properties of glyphosate, the health problems caused by genetically modified crops, and the importance of maintaining gut health, where he still devotes his efforts. But I digress. The law is set up to protect pharmaceutical companies' financial interests by purchasing patents. A proprietary copyright law journal in 2020 (Gurgula, 2020) reported, "One of the reasons that typically leads to high (drug) prices is strategic patenting employed by pharmaceutical companies." One publicized example is CellPro, a Seattle startup company that developed a stem cell separation device, for which it secured FDA approval, lost a patent battle with Johns Hopkins University, Baxter Healthcare Corp, and Becton, Dickinson & Co., and went bankrupt (Bar-Shalom & Cook-Deegan, 2002). Thus, we never saw its presence on the market in the highly competitive field of who owns what. And those that already own the most end up owning more.

Drug development can be an expensive and drawn-out process. Some of the most well-known cancer treatments were initially derived from natural sources, but the end results seem quite far removed. In the early 1960s, for example, two researchers from the US Department of Agriculture identified extracts obtained from the bark of the pacific yew tree that were found to inhibit the growth of certain cancer cells (Baguley, 2002; DeVita & Chu, 2008; Mandal, 2023; Zwawiak & Zaprutko, 2014). The active compound from Taxus brevifolia, paclitaxel, was isolated and run through clinical trials over the next two decades, in an attempt to develop acceptable drug delivery systems. Poly-sciences, Inc. found a more common precursor, 10-deacetylbaccatin III, from the common yew, Taxus baccata, which was then chemically synthesized to paclitaxel. Phyton Catalytic developed the cell culture and Bristol-Myers Squibb trademarked Taxol, which was finally approved in 1994 by the FDA. It was 32 years in the making, but well worth their time, being the best-selling cancer drug ever manufactured and generating 1.6 billion dollars per year for Bristol-Myers Squibb.

In 1913, the American Society for the Control of Cancer was formed by ten physicians and five businessmen, John D. Rockefeller included, who funded the endeavor. Their reported agenda was to raise the awareness of cancer. In 1914, the Society printed and mailed out pamphlets to 14,000 people with "facts" about cancer, and by 1922 their budget went into educating the public, which primarily was targeted at debunking natural remedies, while establishing cancer clinics where only allopathic diagnosis and surgical treatments were allowed, followed by radiation and eventually chemotherapy. Rockefeller continued to donate large sums of money to the organization and in the late 1920s pamphlets were released on the "Danger Signals of Cancer" and "What Every Woman Should Know About Cancer." In 1945, the Society was reorganized and its name was changed to the American Cancer Society.

Meanwhile, during the Second World War, the US military was experimenting with chemical warfare agents and developed nitrogen mustard, which effectively killed or sickened those who came into contact with it. Medical examination of survivors showed their lymphocytes had been dramatically reduced, and in 1942, the first chemotherapeutic drug, mustine (HN2), was developed by Yale University School of Medicine to treat lymphoma. While mustine is no longer in use due to its excessive toxicity, HN2 became the basis of other nitrogen mustard chemotherapeutic agents. Soon afterwards, in 1947, aminopterin was synthetically derived from pterin, an enzyme inhibitor that competes for the folic acid binding site of dihydrofolate reductase, causing the depletion of nucleotide precursors that inhibit DNA, RNA, and protein synthesis. This drug was capable of bringing about remissions in leukemia. By 1956, methotrexate was used in the treatment of choriocarcinoma, a malignant form of uterine cancer.

A decade later, chemotherapy became a mainstay of treatment; present-day cytotoxic drugs are being manufactured that more specifically target individual cancer cells; more recent pharmaceutical agents have been developed to reduce the side effects caused by other pharmaceuticals, and there are even pharmacological agents aimed at overcoming resistance to pharmacological agents. Despite the billions of dollars that are poured into cancer research annually, cancer deaths number approximately ten million per year globally. Costs of cancer treatment are incredibly high, often over $100,000 per patient. Chemotherapy generates about one quarter of the net revenues for the major pharmaceutical companies, and sales of cancer drugs increased 70 percent from 2010 to 2019 (Meyers, *et al.* 2021). Chemotherapeutic drugs now generate well over 100 billion dollars per year. It's hard to tell if there is a cancer epidemic or a chemotherapy epidemic.

Still, despite the fact that natural remedies have been touted as potentially dangerous, various statistics show that more than half of those diagnosed with cancer in the Western world use natural medicine as part of their healing regimen. A recent survey (Blevins Primeau, 2023) reported that 70 percent of cancer patients use complementary or alternative medicine. (Interestingly, a third of them did not tell their oncologists.) Our treatments, while outside mainstream acceptance, are not more right or wrong, they just differ in approach. Instead of poisoning the body to destroy cancer cells, we address the underlying patterns while tending to mental, emotional, and spiritual dimensions of care. It's also important to note that some patients live with cancer cells and tumorous growths for a great many years without reducing the quality of their lives.

Cancer may not need to be as intimidating as the prevailing mindset would have us believe, but because of the public awareness campaigns over the last hundred years, a cancer diagnosis has become highly charged with emotion. Cancer is just an innocuous word until we impart it with our own meaning:

"My sister was born under the sign of Cancer; that's why she feels so deeply."

"I thought a mole on my back was cancer. Turns out it was just a mole."

"The most significant change in my life occurred as a result of my cancer diagnosis."

Imagine receiving the diagnosis yourself, and complete the following sentences:

"If I get cancer, I will..."

"If I don't get cancer, I will..."

Ideally, the answers will be the same or at least similar, and I hope will have something to do with love.

We are told in the Classics that all healing comes from the Heart, and I concur with this sweeping statement, even where cancer is concerned. We've all run across stories of miraculous cures that came about from raising consciousness with no need for chemical remedies. There are many examples of those who have survived their cancer diagnoses without resorting to chemotherapy. Not everyone with cancer needs chemotherapy or is going to die from their cancer. Like Zach Bush said, nobody ever came down with cancer because they were deficient in essential components found only in chemotherapy. This view, however, is not popular, nor is it the norm. Cells that have lost their inner regulatory control circulate through our systems all the time, and our immune cells take care of them. As with any other disease process, the higher the energetic frequency one is able to hold, the greater the capacity to modify one's cellular response and allow the body's intrinsic ability to heal itself. A healthy immune system, the result of a healthy mind that's not in conflict, is continuously removing these cancerous cells from circulation.

Even with a full-blown cancer diagnosis along with conventional treatments, cures are possible. A physician I knew was diagnosed with stage four lung cancer, and after finishing all of the chemotherapeutic approaches that her oncological team had to offer was written off to fly home and spend the remainder of her days in a hospice. Chemo didn't destroy the cancer, and she was left paralyzed, riddled with tumors in her brain and spine. But something happened on the way to palliative care. It was something about the way her son fearlessly stood up for her during the boarding process and treated her with respect and dignity as she was wheeled onto the plane. She experienced for the first time ever that life was unconditionally good and there was nothing to fear. She felt the power of love wash through her body and mind, and rode home in bliss, knowing all was well and she was soon to die. But she didn't. Not for another 25 years. She went into full remission and resumed full ambulation, with a powerful story to tell of the healing power of redemption, of fully accepting ourselves as we are, without resistance or avoidance. With dignity, even if we are facing death. True healing comes when you no longer have the need to fix things, as there is no longer any conflict.

While I am not a cancer specialist, I have worked with patients diagnosed with numerous cancers who were convinced that complications from chemotherapy and radiation were responsible for the development of later cancers. I have worked with patients who opted to address the internal environment with Chinese medicine and avoid chemotherapy and radiation altogether. One in particular was severely scolded by his oncological surgeon when he told her he didn't want to participate in their fear-based approach or take the drugs they insisted he needed to stay alive. His surgeon warned him: "You *should* be scared. You should be *very afraid*. This cancer is going to kill you." In this type of environment, shrouded in fear and worry, it takes a special kind of discipline to cultivate optimism, but he did. When he chose to trust the ability to heal without chemotherapy or radiation, they had nothing left to offer him. I was quite shocked when I tried to find an acupuncturist in his local area to work with him, and nobody would take him on. One very reputable practitioner said he was only comfortable working with cancer patients who were receiving oncological care, and would be happy to focus on reducing the side effects of the medication, but didn't think it was a good idea to rely on Chinese medicine alone. Such are the common biases around cancer, in both conventional and natural medicine. Each of us has the choice to believe in the power of illness, or be liberated from this paradigm. I choose to see the power of wellness in all patients, regardless of their medical diagnosis or treatments they choose, and the healing power of their Hearts seem to respond. He is still alive and well; thriving in fact, and refuses to view himself as a "survivor" any more than you or me.

Etiology

The formation of cancers is varied and complex; their development can't be nailed down to any particular external agent or internal response, as all levels participate.

- External causes include a myriad of environmental factors such as industrial toxins, dietary toxins from common agricultural practices, medications, infectious diseases, and alcohol and tobacco use. Lest we be overwhelmed by our toxic environment, the body is meant to be able to filter out and rid itself of these otherwise potentially harmful exogenous pathogenic factors. Our genome is changing due to these influences brought about by industry, technology, and the readily available information flooding our Jing-well portals, while we are becoming increasingly more sedentary because we never have to leave our chairs to attain information. Our DNA, which tries to mutate to adapt to environmental shifts, hasn't evolved enough yet to accommodate these changes, which would usually take a couple of generations.

- Internal causes are multifactorial, including all levels of Qi:
  - Wei Qi: We must have strong immune systems which are capable of recognizing and eliminating disordered cells. Wei Qi maintains the integrity of the external, the gut, and how our immune cells respond to non-self cells. A healthy immune system, under the domain of the Lung and Liver, evolves as we and our environment change. The Wei Qi ascertains which cells are to be eliminated and which are to be retained. And for this crucial function, it must know, from the marrow outward, who we are and what we are about in order that it may maintain appropriate boundaries.
  - Ying Qi: Primarily belongs to the Spleen and Heart. Long-term stress can disrupt the Qi mechanism. We may not know how to honor ourselves, and get lost in worldly demands or imbalanced relational dynamics. This type of internal conflict might express itself in the cells' loss of internal regulation, which is maintained via negative feedback. The Ying level also includes Blood, which contains our emotional makeup. Internal dysregulation often stems from unacknowledged emotional conflicts that can produce toxic effects in the Blood. The Luo Mai confront issues carried in the Blood lines. Cancers associated with the middle Jiao may derive from things the body can't properly digest, whether xenobiotics, chemical toxins, or psychic issues.
  - Yuan Qi: Belongs to the collective rather than an individual's sense of self alone. It represents the survival of the species more than survival of the individual. Paradoxically, however, it also carries our

fundamental constitutional level, our initial starting point carried out by the Kidneys and San Jiao. Who we inherently are can't be separated from the whole or the challenges we will encounter in life. Conflicts that remain unconsciously held in the shadow realm are under the domain of the Kidneys. All cancers involve the proliferative tissue carried in our Essence. When Jing becomes unstable, it can literally forget how to cease proliferating, causing the Yang Qi to grow out of control. Lower Jiao presentations arise from proliferative tissues in the ovary, uterus, testicles, and prostate. We may also inherit a certain susceptibility to gene repair defects like BRA1 or BRA2 in breast and ovarian tissues; however, the presence of the genes is less important than the epigenetic programming responsible for turning them on and off, which equates to how we live our lives. Studies have shown that the biofield, the underlying Qi one inhabits, determines whether or not cancer genes will be expressed (Rubik *et al.*, 2015). Working with the Eight Extraordinary Vessels allows us to tap into the constitutional level and help the individual resolve hidden conflicts held in the Jing. As Jing declines through the process of living and aging, we must protect the Curious Organs, which allow for evolution and adaptation. The Gallbladder, for example, is able to contain Heat to keep it from spreading to the breast and brain. The divergent meridians also hold pathogens in latency. Here, pathologic Qi is displaced from the Wei Qi level, becoming trapped in the density of Jing. The individual doesn't have to deal with the issue presently, and can go about their life while Jing holds the evil at bay. Meanwhile, the Heat of Wei Qi simmers in the depths, potentially damaging the DNA. As we age or our Jing declines, the pathogenic factors and our response to them can no longer be contained, and they may seep out into the circulation, resulting in a myriad of potential manifestations. Based on the strength of the Jing, Blood, Ying, Jin/ Ye, Yang Qi, or other medium of holding, we will have to determine whether the body has the resources to release the pathogen, or if we should attempt to facilitate its holding in latency.

All of the above factors can contribute to the depletion of Spleen and Kidney Qi, while patterns of Dampness, Phlegm, Qi stagnation, and Blood stasis may conglomerate into tumors, and Toxic Heat may cause the Jing to flare out of control. We are becoming more predisposed to cancers today, not just due to environmental factors, but because we don't have adequate Yin to support the demands of excess Yang; we are stressed and our nerves are fried, leaving us with chronic Lung Yin deficiency. We bear the collective grief for the effects of greed out of control, planetary demise, and the inability to perpetuate ourselves. Our ways of being have been scrambled, and we haven't been able to catch up with whatever direction we are headed. Perhaps this is all preparation for a new reality, though, no longer governed by fear, separation, and greed, but by unity and faith in the power of nature to heal us by restoring the goodness of humanity.

Pathogenesis

Genetic signaling is encoded within the Jing, but is influenced by other epigenetic factors. There is an underlying "push" of Yuan Qi that leads to cellular division, a function of Yang Qi. In a harmonious environment, normal genetic signaling is encoded within the DNA, allowing cells to respond harmoniously to this push and grow in a controlled manner. Depending on the cell's specific function, each has also been pre-programmed for its own demise, a process referred to as apoptosis. As fingers and toes develop from hand and foot buds, apoptosis halts the cells that would otherwise have become webs between the digits from developing. When underlying patterns of imbalance cause this signaling to go awry, the programmed cellular death, the "off" switch, malfunctions. In the presence of Toxic Heat, the Yin "stop" message isn't received, and the cells proliferate rapidly, growing out of control and damaging the Yuan Qi. Jing flares out of control, no longer rooted in its primary directive to be itself. As you can see, cancer isn't the root, but a branch symptom of an imbalance that causes the cells to hyperproliferate. The root is an underlying conflict expressing itself within the cells and causing them to lose their regulatory control. The Yang message doesn't turn off, and the cells go rogue, forgetting their natural function and original cellular identity. They become isolated and cut off from cellular communication within the rest of the body. Once these damaged cells fail to keep their proper place in the bodily community, they lose the ability to provide fuel for and repair themselves. Now they have to go out and feed off other bodily fuel sources.

The remedy

Perhaps destruction isn't our only option. These cells aren't evil, but are cut-off fragments that have lost sight of the whole of which they are a part. Much of the healing work we do in this medicine is to integrate and welcome the fragmented parts back into ourselves. We know that when cancer cells reconnect and join with healthy surrounding cells, the thing we call cancer disappears. It is very challenging to find research that supports positive cellular behavior, and doesn't only focus on the aggressive tendencies of cancer cells. However, Mark Frattini, MD, PhD, an expert on blood cancers, said in an article on drug resistant cancers, "The problem is that cancer is smarter than drugs that target specific pathways." He along with other researchers at New York-Presbyterian/Columbia University Irving Medical Center have found that cancer cells can regain control of their growth and return to a normal state (Can we make cancer cells normal again?, 2017). They haven't figured out precisely how, however. As suggested above, instead of rejecting and killing our brokenness, another option might be to befriend it. Then if the cells can't be repaired and incorporated back into the whole, they will remove themselves via apoptosis because their Righteous Qi is intact. Weizman Institute of Sciences published a study in *Cell* (Shir Itai *et al.*, 2024), validating that when immune cells join forces, cancer therapy is more effective.

Patients predisposed to or diagnosed with cancers would be well advised to look at dietary and lifestyle factors first, eliminating toxic substances like nicotine and alcohol, and removing sweets, refined carbohydrates, and preservatives from their diet. The bulk of their diet should come from organic fruits and vegetables, especially bitter greens, which clear Heat and Fire toxins, but should avoid cruciferous vegetables that cluster, as they can bind the Qi. They would benefit from drinking raw vegetable juices like wheat grass, which clears Fire toxins and can induce Cold. The basis of life comes from the sea, and phytoplanktons like blue-green algae, chlorella, and chlorophyll can help bring the enlivening properties of oxygenation and nutrients to repair damaged cells. Seaweed also softens hard masses. The saltiness of silkworms, Bai Jiang Can, allows them to enter the Jing level to subdue Yang, and expel Wind, Phlegm, and Heat. Nuts and nut milks tonify the Lung Qi, as do compact fruits. Watercress can be used for Kidney Fire, and dandelions for Liver Fire. Ai Ye and Qing Hao can target Damp and fermented environments, which become acidic and promote carcinogenic growths. These dietary practices can all help the body become more alkaline. Cancer, which loves acidity, also loves sugar, and another alkaline delivery process is to mix five tablespoons of maple syrup with two tablespoons of baking soda. Warm over very low heat and stir until it starts to foam. Refrigerate and take one to two teaspoonfuls per day. The sugar will go to the cancer cells and deliver the alkaline bicarbonate.

Our diagnostic skills challenge us to remain on the lookout for deficiencies in Jing, Qi, and Blood, and the emergence of Toxic Heat or swellings. Weakness in the Jing almost always correlates with a lost sense of our true nature. Our Kidneys should be still and quiet, as stillness leads to the ability to store. The deeper we query who we are and why we are here, the more likely the Jing is to recall its function. We are here on purpose, and if our destiny still eludes us, perhaps a challenge like cancer can cause us to remember. This is why many people acknowledge that their cancer diagnosis woke them up to the gift of this very life, and they began to recognize the effects of harsh and unloving attitudes toward themselves. Disease can be an invitation into the truth contained within, and cancer can be a loud wake-up call. As we go within and learn to explore the deepest aspects of ourselves, we have to reckon with our wills, the spirit of the Kidneys. Shen animates and fulfills the purpose of our lives. If we aren't following the path of our curriculum to achieve completion in this life, we often end up exhausting our Jing, which then begins to decay. Part of our job should be to help patients de-program corrosive messages in the Jing by encouraging them to look at any internal conflicts in their lives. Depending on the types of carcinoma, and the patterns that underly them, different questions might lead them toward the source. What is missing in your life? What have you been unable to reproduce in your life? Are there any past events that you still lament? Failure to go to the root and meet this challenge may also be why the recurrence rate of cancer is so high.

Reproductive cancers are on the rise, partly because of the abundance of environmental xenoestrogens; these overgrowths may also have metaphysical roots in issues pertaining to creativity, the Palace of the Child. The Bao consolidates the mystery of life by wrapping up the Jing and weaving the energy of Heaven and Earth together to create something new. In a corrosive environment, all of the elements are there to produce something new which is yet not conducive to life. Also, the conversion of Yuan Qi to Ying Qi may become obstructed, giving rise to uncontrolled abnormal growth via the Blood.

First, we have to discern where the Heat is found. Which pulses are the most rapid, and what part of the tongue shows the most redness? The underside of the tongue may also show branching sublingual veins in the area associated with the carcinogenic lesion. Phlegmy nodules at the base of the tongue can also be associated with attempts to keep the Heat at bay. Heat spreads and translocates by nature, and it is this mechanism that is responsible for the aggressiveness of cancers, regardless of the cause. The energies of both the Lung and the Heart can spread into the uterus. Toxins can localize in the Bao, and become tumorous.

We then have to ask how weak or strong the patient is. If they are strong enough, we can work with clearing Fire toxins. Fire toxins can be complicated by Damp Heat which can stifle the Heat to keep the Fire from traveling upward, Blood Heat, and Phlegm Heat. When Damp Heat is present, we need to work with disinhibiting the bowels. Using Ll 6, St 40, SI 7, SJ 5, GB 36, and UB 57 can help clear Fire toxins and release the bowels. You may also bleed Ll 11, St 36, Du 9, and Du 14.

If the person is weak, perhaps they aren't capable of challenging their beliefs, changing their diet, modifying their lifestyle, divorcing an abusive spouse, and so on, and perhaps our present strategy will be to help the patient live with the tumor and help put it into remission. We may need to tonify the Qi with herbs like Bai Zhu, Da Zao, and Shan Yao and nourish Yin with Han Lian Cao, Nu Zhen Zi, and Gui Ban, while inducing Cold with minerals like Shi Gao and Han Shui Shi to maintain latency.

Carcinomas don't always have their origins in Heat, however. Weakness of the Spleen can hinder the strength of the Wei Qi and cause Dampness. Cold and Dampness can develop into Blood stasis, and produce tumorous swellings for which the Fire School might recommend Si Ni Tang, especially when patients are cold and have lost weight. Cancerous cells can also combine with microbial agents like viral pathogens, the nature of which is Cold. Viruses like HPV like to live in the uterus, for example. Now the immune system will be challenged to deal with both the virus and cancerous cells. When the Wei Qi isn't strong enough to rid the exogenous pathogenic factor, it often travels to the Bladder where it can translocate to the Shu points and enter into other organs. Stagnation causes the body to detoxify at a slower rate, which can also lead to metastasis. Cancers can also spread via the lymph or blood. Here we may want to use Divergent or Luo treatments. Lymph node involvement also pertains to Jin fluids, so our treatments will include regulating fluid metabolism. Ye has its relationship with the bone and marrow, and Liver metastasis with the Blood. Da Huang can help purge and clear stagnation at the Blood level, combined with Yu Jin. Sea vegetables can help soften hardness due to stagnation involving the Kidneys, where Phlegmy masses have developed. The Spleen then takes on its special function as remonstrator, letting the Emperor know an error has been made; and the Spleen will begin the process of digesting itself to dissolve the tumor.

The Shen, via the Blood, has to penetrate into the uterus. If one is disengaged from their origin, Ren 4, the gateway to the source, can invigorate the reproductive organs. As the front Mu point of the Small Intestine, it can also address issues concerning lack of control, or where patients are feeling deeply inadequate. Since Ren 4 represents where the three Yin leg channels come together, it is prone to Yin stasis. But you don't want to needle Ren 4 when the uterus is the site of active cancer.

Reproductive cancers often relate back to the Da Bao above or Dai Mai below. GB 22 can open what's bound in the chest; GB 41 can liberate unprocessed grief and unshed tears; GB 27 can help release the ancestral pillars, and GB 28 can help let go of any toxicity that one hasn't been able to set free. When one seems to be stuck in a clouded stupor, seeing the world the same way without change, we can work with the Jing Well points of Fire, Pc 8, and Water, Ki 1, to help resuscitate Yang, to open consciousness and allow new perspectives.

Herbally we want to use bitter herbs that descend. Xia Ku Cao usually goes to the eyes and throat, but when processed with vinegar it develops a descending property. It is the same with Pu Gong Yin; when processed with vinegar, it can descend. Bai Mao Gen is often used, and Zhi Mu and Huang Bai can clear Heat, while nourishing Yin and protecting fluids. Huang Jing can be used concurrently to nourish Yin, strengthen Jing, and tonify Qi. Mushrooms can also enhance immunity; reishi has an affinity for the Liver; shitake and maitake for the Spleen; black mu er for the Kidneys; and lion's mane mushrooms for the brain and mucosal tissues. When we tonify the Yin, Qi, and Blood, tumor sizes may initially increase before shrinking. We aren't assessing improvement based on the size of the carcinogenic lesion, but on how well the patterns are changing. Is the Toxic Heat lessening? Is the Wei Qi improving? Are the Kidneys getting stronger?

We also must enhance the Wei Qi and tonify the Lungs. The Lungs, human gills that resonate with heavenly Qi, deal with issues surrounding life and death. As we inspire, we are filled with Heaven. As we exhale, we are to relinquish as many earthly attachments as we can so we may connect with the canopy of Heaven. When one receives a cancer diagnosis, all of their hopes and dreams of the future are at stake, and all they are left with is the immediacy of their own existence. This can cause the ultimate surrender, which tonifies the Lungs more than any herb or needle can accomplish on its own.

Our immune system is always taking care of pre-cancerous and cancerous cells which are a part of life. Jing proliferates. And even though it is the Yuan Qi, the very sense of who we are that has gone rogue, we tend to depersonalize cancer. When we see the cancer as separate from us, then we can go to war against it. It's much easier to kill this thing that's not seen as me. And yet, it is. Perhaps this is one reason why we can't win the "war against cancer." Another approach is to open up to it and meet this entity as an aspect of self, and invite it in. How did it become cut off and alienated? Instead of banishing it, we can become very present with it (Ki 9) and ask what it needs. Does it need to be welcomed back (St 9)? Each manifestation will have its own characteristics, so can't be approached with pre-established protocols.

A vast chasm exists between this mythopoetic view, and the absolute view of Western science. In one, the very meaning of our lives determines the outcome, and in the other, eradication of the evil is the only thing that matters. And in this case destruction of the evil Qi also destroys the righteous Qi. Oncology does what it does well, but carries some of the trappings of weaponization, where chemical arms seek to eradicate everything in their path, good and bad alike, in attempting to gain control over life. If an advanced life form looked in at our present conventional treatment of cancer, it might appear rather barbaric. The state of one's consciousness isn't taken into consideration; just find the enemy and kill it. This may be viewed as a manifestation of an outmoded and dis-eased thought system that deems some things good and others bad, and seeks to destroy the evil, which always belongs to the depersonalized "other." We have a societal agreement that all cancer is bad, and must be eradicated at all cost. Only from a state of fear would anyone agree to bathe every cell in their body in poison, with the whisper of a promise that maybe they won't die. Well, guess what? Someday they will.

I'm obviously highlighting a very one-sided view of the treatment of cancer here. I don't think everyone should adopt the view that all chemo is bad either, and should be avoided at all costs. But I hope that if more people question the assumptions we have been living under, we will find our way back to the center, where we can make more mindful decisions about our therapeutic course of action, and nature will help restore us to harmony. If we are to believe the *Ling Shu*, which I hope all readers do, the Shen are the root cause of all disease. Shen are the motivating force of Qi. All disease, cancer included, is a Qi imbalance, and therefore rooted in a spiritual imbalance. Therefore, caring for the spirit should be a clinician's primary role.

The *Tao te Ching* abounds with phrases that can help us challenge the unquestioned narrative of patriarchal control trying to dominate nature:

> Only when we aren't trying to gain power do we have power... When people no longer trust themselves, they begin to depend upon authority... The greatest wisdom may appear childish... Only when we leave nature alone do we find harmony... Trying to control outcomes is like handling the master carpenter's tools; chances are you'll cut yourself... Those who try to control, go against the direction of the Tao... If you aren't afraid of dying, there is nothing you can't achieve...

Our job is to promote health, and healing doesn't always mean living longer. Sometimes death is the greatest healer.

Radiotherapy

Radiation therapy utilizes high doses of radiation to damage the DNA of cancer cells and kill them. Both X-rays and proton radiation therapies are localized, and aim the beams directly at the affected tissues. Radiation oncology may be employed in the early stages of cancer or after it has started to spread. Therapies may be used by themselves or in conjunction with chemotherapy. After radiation treatment, patients experience fatigue and skin changes from the burning properties of radiation. Other side effects include hair loss, nausea, vomiting, weight loss, headache, blurred vision, loss of concentration, and memory problems. Patients also report local burning sensations, and loss of use of the affected area as surrounding healthy tissues and organs can be damaged due to the intensity of Heat. One of the major drawbacks of radiation therapy is that it can increase the risk of developing other cancers later. When our patients are receiving radiotherapy, treatments will be supportive, and aimed at reducing the side effects by clearing Heat, and tonifying Yin, Qi, and Blood.

Chemotherapeutic agents

Chemotherapy is considered a "clearing" strategy used to combat cancer. Antineoplastic drugs refer to a group of pharmaceuticals with chemical properties that produce cytotoxic effects, preventing the growth of neoplasms as well as normal tissue growth. This class of drugs, which has multiple subcategories, targets DNA and specific metabolic steps required in cellular replication. These cytotoxic drugs are absorbed by rapidly growing cells in order to inhibit DNA replication. The epithelial linings of the bowel, bladder, lungs, reproductive organs, hair, and bone marrow are particularly susceptible, and side effects will thus include nausea, vomiting, diarrhea, constipation, hair loss, mouth sores, and immune dysfunction.

While these therapies often decrease tumor growth, reduction in tumor growth doesn't necessarily correlate with increased survival rates, as the drugs are not intending to address the chronic excess conditions that give rise to the overgrowths. Their mechanism of action is to weaken or stifle the Yuan Qi, inhibiting the conversion of Yuan Qi to Ying Qi, which then disrupts Kidney Yang's transformation to Spleen Qi, as well as Kidney Yin's ability to generate Liver Blood. Patients whose Jing is too weak should be wary of jumping into chemotherapeutic treatments. Check the Kidney Yin pulse to see if it has the strength to move the chemo drugs out. If the person dosen't have the ability to process the chemo, our treatment principles should be to build Yin to hold the cancer in latency. One month of building Yin reserves might help them handle the effects of the chemo. Further, if the Liver pulse is tight, there may be too much Qi stagnation to allow them to detox properly, and their Liver must be harmonized in order to recover.

Some chemotherapeutic agents are Cold therapies that inhibit Yang Qi actions, making patients feel cold, and some antineoplastics have Hot effects which damage the Yin, causing symptoms such as hair loss and mouth sores. Many do both, as freezing and burning are equally effective at destroying the Jing, and individual responses to both will vary. Some agents cause nausea and vomiting; check the Stomach pulse to see if it descends from the superficial to moderate level. If not, Ren 12 and 13 can help the Stomach Qi descend. Some cytotoxic agents impact the bowels resulting in either diarrhea or constipation. While diarrhea is annoying, it is not problematic for a couple of days. We want them to be able to release toxicity by moving the bowels. Constipation is more concerning, however, and if they aren't moving the bowels daily, treatment principles must include helping the bowels to purge (St 25, St 37, UB 36) so they can rid their body of the harmful effects of these toxic pharmaceutical agents. Our treatments will always address the symptoms of the chemotherapy, while supporting the immune system. We should always support the upright Qi and tonify the Spleen in patients receiving chemotherapy. Astragalus can increase stamina and strength, reduce fatigue, strengthen the immune system, and reduce nausea. It is advisable to tonify the Qi, Blood, and Yin before, during, and after chemotherapy, calm the Shen, and provide whatever physical or emotional support the person needs. Since most poisonous substances like chemotherapy end up inducing Cold and Blood stasis, we often have to warm, invigorate the Blood, and address symptoms like peripheral neuropathy, for which Ba Xie and Ba Feng points can be helpful.

Alkylating agents directly impact DNA linkage to inhibit cellular reproduction. They consist of:

- nitrogen mustards (Chlorambucil, Cyclophosphamide, Ifosfamide, Mechlorethamine, Melphalen)
- nitrogen mustard analogues: bendamustine (Belrapzo, Bendeka, Vivimusta)
- nitrosoureas (Carmustine, Aranose, Chlorozoticin, Ethylnitrosourea, Fotemustine, Lomustine, Nimustine, Neuromedin U, Ranimustine, Semustine, Streptozocin)
- alkylsulfonates (Busulfan)
- triazines (Dacarbazine, Temozolomide)
- etholenimines (Altretamine, Thiotepa).

Alkylating agents disrupt cellular division, a Yang function at the Yuan Qi level, by damaging the RNA or DNA, a process which inhibits Yang Qi's ability to convert Yuan Qi to Ying Qi, or Jing to Blood. Cyclophosphamide is a nitrogen mustard that exerts its effects through alkylation. This cross-links DNA so it can't replicate, and is toxic to lymphocytes. Alkylating agents attempt to use Heat to move the localized Heat response. Common side effects include nausea, vomiting, hair loss, taste changes, numbness, weakness, arthralgia, and cognitive impairments like memory loss, difficulty concentrating, and depression. Bone marrow suppression can lead to lowered immunity, severe blood disorders, anemia, leukopenia, and thrombocytopenia.

Because of the clearing nature of the mustards, we need to nourish Lung and Stomach Yin with herbs like Mai Men Dong and Tian Men Dong, and Shi Hu. Herbs which address food stasis can help build the Yin and help digestion. Clear Heat as appropriate.

Platinum agents

- Carboplatin (Paraplatin)
- Cisplatin (Platinol)
- Oxaliplatin (Eloxatin)
- Nedaplatin (Aqupla)

These directly impact DNA linkage to inhibit cellular reproduction. Platinum is a metal with cooling properties that damages the DNA, primarily interfering with the Yuan Qi level, and secondarily with channel and organ function. These drugs severely impact the Jing as well as functions which stem from or relate to the Kidneys. This means that the Spleen will have difficulty making Blood, and Wei Qi will be weakened. In order to best support a patient who is taking this drug, it is imperative to nourish fluids via the San Jiao mechanism, and to move the bowels. There has to be a way for the toxicity to exit the body, which can be done effectively through stool excretion. Further, peridot elixir can help chelate the platinum out of the body. It is also vital to nourish the Sea of Blood after treatment due to the impact of the drugs on all three levels of Qi. Additionally, it is important to supplement Qi, Yin, and Yang via herbal medicine and acupuncture. The Three Triangles acupuncture treatment (Ren 12, St 36; Ren 13, Pc 6; Ren 10, St 25) can be very effective to manage side effects on the day of chemotherapy delivery, and on the days when the side effects of the chemotherapy treatment are flaring. When patients experience peripheral neuropathy, this indicates deficient Liver Blood, which will tend to become stagnant. Ji Xue Teng can help open the channels, relax the tendons, tonify Blood, and eliminate Stasis.

Antimetabolites

- 6-mercaptopurine (Purinethol)
- Azacitidine, 5-fluorouracil (Adrucil)
- Capecitabine (Xeloda)
- Cladribine (Mavenclad, Leustatin)
- Clofarabine (Clolar)
- Cytarabine (Depocyt)
- Decitabine (Dacogen)
- Floxuridine (FUDR)
- Fludarabine (Fludara, Oforta)
- Gemcitabine (Gemzar, Infugem)
- Hydroxyurea (Hydrea, Siklos, Mylocel, Droxia)
- Mercaptopurine (Purinethol)
- Methotrexate (Otrexup, Rheumatrex, Trexall, Rasuvo)
- Nelarabine (Arranon)
- Pemetrexed (Alimta, Pemfexy)

- Pentostatin, pralatrexate (Folotyn)
- Thioguanine (Tabloid)
- Trifluridine/tipiracil (Lonsurf)

These drugs inhibit the synthesis of purine (Adenine and Guanine) or pyrimidine (Cytosine and Thymine), the nitrogenous bases that make up DNA strands. They block DNA replication, resulting in cellular death. They are used to treat carcinomas of the breast, bowel, skin, stomach, esophagus, and pancreas. They irritate the epithelial tissues and can thus cause side effects such as nausea, vomiting, diarrhea, constipation, loss of appetite, and mouth sores. They may also induce numbness, pain, and tingling of the arms, legs, fingers, and toes, and cause bone marrow suppression. While these herbs act by blocking the foundation of Jing, we can support patients on antimetabolites by nourishing Stomach and Lung Yin and supporting Kidney Essence with herbs like Han Lian Cao, Nu Zhen Zi, and Huang Jing.

Topoisomerase inhibitors
Topoisomerase is an important component in DNA organization and cellular reproduction. These drugs block a step that generates strand breaks in the cellular cycle, leading to apoptotic death of the cell. Antineoplastic topoisomerase inhibitors are a synthetic version of camptothecin, which is extracted from the bark of the Camptotheca aluminata tree (Belotecan, Irinotecan, Topotecan, Etoposide, Mitoxantrone, Teniposide, Camptosar, Enhertu, Hycamtin, Onivyde, Sacituzumab, Trodelvy). Used to treat colorectal, pancreatic, urothelial, ovarian, breast, gastric, lung, and cervical cancers, these drugs cause the DNA strand to break, killing the cells. Like most other cytotoxic drugs, side effects include nausea, vomiting, constipation, diarrhea, heartburn, loss of appetite, mouth sores, back pain, abdominal pain, headache, weakness, fatigue, dry skin and eyes, and altered taste sensations. Again, we will support the Essence and tonify Yin. Descend Qi when rebellious. Open the bowels if constipated, and clear Heat when Heat signs are pronounced.

Mitotic inhibitors

- Docetaxel (Docefrez, Taxotere)

- Eribulin (Havalen)
- Paclitaxel (Taxol, Abraxane, Onxol)
- Vincristine (Vincasar)
- Teniposide (Vumon)
- Etoposide (VePesid, Toposar)
- Vinblastine (Velban)
- Vincristine sulfate (Marqibo)
- Vinorelbine (Navelbine)
- Cabazitaxel (Jevtana)
- Ixabepilone (Ixempra)
- Etoposide (Etopophos)
- Estramustine (Emcyt)

These are antimicrotubule agents that intend to slow or stop the growth of cancer cells. They enter the DNA and interrupt the spindle cells, virtually causing the cancer cells to develop their own cancer, thus intending to interfere with their uncontrolled growth. This impacts the DNA of all body cells, and can thus induce cancer in healthy cells of the body. The resulting criss-crossing effect of the spindle cells is like Shao Yang disease. Side effects include nausea, vomiting, diarrhea, mouth sores, flushing, numbness, tingling and burning of the hands and feet, muscle and joint pain, dizziness, drowsiness, brain fog, and hair loss. Here we can help to protect the Gallbladder with Qiang Hao formulas.

Anti-tumor antibiotics

- Daunorubicin (Cerubidine, Daunoxome)
- Doxorubicin (Adriamycin, Doxil)
- Epirubicin (Ellence)
- Idarubicin (Idamycin)
- Valrubicin (Valstar)
- Bleomycin (Blenoxane)
- Dactinomycin (Cosmegen)
- Mitomycin (Jelmyto, Mutamycin, Mitosol)
- Mitoxantrone (Novantrone)

- Pentostatin (Nipent)

These anti-tumor antibiotics cause breakage in the DNA strands. While antibiotics are usually Cold, these are cultured from the strep bacteria and are chelated to hydrogen chloride, an acid, which renders these treatments hot and warming. They will cause the body to heat up, and the patient will feel hot and feverish, and prone to dryness. They are used for aggressive conditions, such as lymphocytic leukemia, and target the lymphatic system. We can help clear Heat, open the throat, and, if the tongue tip is red, clear Heat in the Heart. Cardiotoxicity is one of the most common long-term side effects of these drugs. Dark sublingual veins will show poor vascular energy, and we may need to move stuck Qi and Blood.

Miscellaneous group of specific cytotoxic pharmaceuticals

- Antracycline tretinoin blocks enzymes needed for cellular growth.
- Arsenic trioxide stops cells from dividing or spreading, but can cause damage to the heart.
- Asparaginase is a bacterial enzyme with antineoplastic effects that can have severe effects on the liver, including hepatic failure.
- Eribulin's cytotoxic effects are due to its inhibition of microtubule function, but it can also cause liver damage.
- Epothilones: ixabelipone (Ixempra) damages cancer cells through tubulin polymerization.
- Mitotane (Lysodren) treats a rare type of carcinoma of the adrenal gland, and produces quite an array of unique side effects.
- Omacetaxine is an mRNA protein translation inhibitor for the treatment of chronic myeloid leukemia.
- Pegaspargase (Oncaspar) targets acute lymphoblastic leukemia.
- Procarbazine (Matulane) is an alkylating agent used to treat Hodgkin's lymphoma.
- Romidepsin and vorinostat are histone deacetylase inhibitors that target cutaneous T-cell lymphomas.

Immunotherapies

While some immunotherapies attempt to suppress overactive immune responses, the immune system must remain strong in order to recover and be able to detoxify after chemotherapy. Certain immunotherapies attempt to modulate immune responses, usually combined with other cytotoxic therapies, to help the immune system recognize and destroy cancer cells. By modulating Wei Qi activity, these therapies are often going to have their effects at the Tai Yang and Yang Ming levels. Side effects include fatigue, coughing, chills, fever, flu-like symptoms, pain, itching, rashes, blisters, dry eyes, headaches, and constipation. Our treatments can help support by clearing Heat, releasing the exterior, and tonifying Qi, Yin, and Blood.

- Interferons are signaling proteins released by host cells to trigger the immune cells to arrest growth and promote apoptosis in viral and cancer cells. Interferon therapy was the first immunotherapeutic drug approved by the FDA. It has since been replaced by other targeted therapies but is still used in conjunction with radiotherapies and chemotherapies.

- Interleukins are a type of cytokine produced by leukocytes and other cells to modulate immune reactions, helping immune cells grow and divide more quickly.

- Monoclonal antibodies like rituximab (Rituxan, MabThera), trastuzumab (Herceptin), alemtuzumab, tositumomab (Bexxar), cetuximab (Erbitux), bevacizumab (Avastin), panitumumab (Vectibix), catumaxomab (Removab), ofatumumab (Arzerra, Kesimpta), ipilimumab (Yervoy), nivolumab (Opdivo), pembrolizumab (Keytruda), pertuzumab (Perjeta), denosumab (Prolia), ibritumomab tiuxetan (Zevalin), brentuximab vedotin (Adcetris), and trastuzumab emtansine (Kadcyla) are used for various conditions including autoimmune diseases and cancers. There are over 500 monoclonal antibodies, which target cancer cells by binding to antigens on the cell surface. Once the monoclonal antibodies attach to the specific cellular protein, they either act on the cells or they trigger the immune system to attack and kill the cancer cells. They are often used in conjunction with other cytotoxic drugs and vascular ablation. Because they intensify immunologic responses, allergic reactions are common. Their side effects include symptoms associated with releasing the exterior: fatigue, feeling sick, fever, chills, flushing, fainting, diarrhea, itchy rashes, and breathlessness.

Estrogen blockers

Certain types of breast cancers grow in response to hormonal stimulation. Estrogens are related to Yin and Blood, with moistening and cooling effects. When estrogens build up in the blood it can produce conditions of Stagnation and Dampness, especially in the absence of Yang to move them. The resulting accumulation can lead to tumorous growths and/or Heat toxins. Aromatase is an enzyme that converts androgens into estrogen. Aromatase inhibitors (Anastrozole, Exemestane, Letrozole) block this conversion, reducing the levels of the active hormone estradiol in the body. This effectively puts the body into a menopausal state, producing side effects like hot flashes, night sweats, vaginal dryness, loss of libido, and joint and muscle pain. This is because the Yin-depleting effects induce dryness, and since Kidney and Liver Yin share the same source, Liver Blood deficiency can fail to nourish the sinews. When Yin isn't sufficient to anchor Yang, empty Heat results.

Selective estrogen receptor modulators (SERM)

Tamoxifen selectively binds to estrogen receptor sites exhibiting both estrogenic and anti-estrogenic effects. It has anti-estrogenic effects on the breast, but estrogenic effects in the endometrium and bone. Tamoxifen increases the risk of developing blood clots, giving rise to deep vein thrombosis, and pulmonary emboli, as well as increasing the likelihood of developing uterine cancers. When the Blood going to the breasts is blocked, the Liver energy will then stagnate or shift downward, giving rise to Dampness and Phlegm accumulation in the uterus. Relax the Liver to reduce stagnation, and use herbs like Yi Yi Ren for Dampness and Hai Zao for Hot Phlegm in the lower Jiao.

Gonadotropin-releasing hormone (GnRH) agonists

- Goserelin (Zoladex)

- Triptorelin, buserelin, leuprolide (Lupron)

These interfere with pituitary signals, which has the effect of suppressing ovarian or testicular production of hormones. Like other hormone-blocking pharmaceuticals, side effects will at least partially be due to the absence of hormones. In women, hot flashes, night sweats, vaginal dryness, loss of sex drive, difficulty sleeping, headaches, dizziness, changes in blood pressure, confusion, loss of coordination, depression, and other mood changes are not uncommon. Depleting both Yin and Yang hormones has drying and Heating effects and can also cause visceral agitation from Yin and Blood deficiency. Tonifying Kidney Essence and Blood, clearing Heat, and nourishing fluids can help patients tolerate the medication and will not reduce the effectiveness of the drugs.

Angiogenesis inhibitors

Cancers need oxygen and nutrition and must establish their own blood supply. Through a process called angiogenesis, when any tissues, tumorous growths included, become deprived of oxygen, they release pro-angiogenic chemicals like vascular endothelial growth factors (VEGF) that initiate new vascular tissue. This allows them to thrive, grow, and spread to other tissues. Angiogenesis-inhibiting drugs—axitinib (Inlyta), bevacizumab (Avastin), cabozantinib (Cometriq), everolimus (Afinitor), lenalidomide (Revlimid), lenvatinib mesylate (Lenvima), pazopanib (Votrient), ramucirumab (Cyramza), regorafenib (Stivarga), sorafenib (Nexavar), sunitinib (Sutent), thalidomide (Synovir, Thalomid), vandetanib (Caprelsa), zif-aflibercept (Zaltrap)—block blood vessel formation by inhibiting different steps involved in the process of vascular proliferation. Some of the side effects of angiotensin inhibitors include blood clots, impaired wound healing, hemorrhage, strokes, heart attacks, hypertension, proteinuria, fatigue, gastrointestinal perforation, fistulas, diarrhea, and hypothyroidism. Asian medicine views abnormal bleeding as caused by Qi vacuity, Blood stasis, or Heat in the Blood. Angiotensin inhibitors seem to share these mechanisms. Inhibiting vascular formation can cause Blood Heat, Blood stasis, and disrupt the Qi mechanism.

We will continue to see new radiological and pharmaceutical developments in the treatment of cancers. If more health care dollars could be siphoned away from pharmaceuticals and put toward fascinating new disciplines like regenerative medicine or biofield science, these advances could revolutionize the health care industry.

We are likely not going to see this ailment eradicated unless we make some radical shifts in how we live life and approach healing. Remember, when someone has a cancer diagnosis, the disease mechanism has already been simmering underground for months or decades, eluding the dictates of their righteous Qi. The highest state of medicine would have addressed the more insidious causative disease factors and helped the patient elevate their Heart mind to live from their true nature, which is based on love. A high percentage of the money spent on cancer prevention research goes toward developing new screening devices, drugs, and vaccines. Healing isn't about the right diagnostic test or chemotherapy. Nor is it only about prevention through quitting smoking or drinking and changing your diet, but uncovering the caustic origins that persist below the level of awareness that keep us from living our highest energetic state. The pulse can detect concealed conflicts even when the conscious mind is in denial. Instead of adopting a "goal-oriented" approach of no longer having cancer, help them shift their mindset to one of healing in this moment. Much of my work with fertility patients focused on helping them let go of the goal of getting pregnant, and instead living a more fertile life. When the Heart-Mind led the way, the Qi followed, and often so did a pregnancy. Focusing on the disease goes against the natural order. Many patients who make it through chemotherapy refer to themselves as "survivors," where their identity has become intertwined with their disease. Yes, they've survived chemotherapy and aren't dead. But it might make more sense to shift their focus away from their cancer history and toward healing their lives.

Do they have any unresolved issues with anyone they've ever known? If the relationships are still alive, they can begin the process of forgiveness and healing to resolve the conflict. They can also work with the spirit of the deceased through their own Shen. We are always trying to find our way back to love, joy, and peace of the Heart. If we are to wholly love ourselves now, we must also include the love of everything that ever happened to us. This doesn't mean we impose a state of gratitude for all of our wounds and traumas, but we can accept that they were necessary parts of our curriculum to bring us where we are today. Do we have compassion for our responses to the difficulties with which we were presented? Whether we believe in God, Heaven, reincarnation, or living a virtuous life with no regrets, rectifying our lives is probably more important than medicating them.

In this way, we continue to realign with the Power of the Way. Pharmaceuticals don't have the power to make us well or to keep us from getting well. When we recognize that it is the state of the Heart-Mind which is most important, our reliance on physical substances to determine the quality of health diminishes. We have this power within us, if only we will discover, utilize, and live it.

Conclusion

My wish for all of us, who give or receive health care, is to return to the healing power of the Heart, which just seems to be so beautifully captured by this wisdom tradition. Many of us have got so far away from nature that we can't even remember the path. Life is a gift freely given, but with certain challenges and responsibilities. It isn't meant to be neat, sanitized, and controlled; we were not created to avoid pain and seek pleasure—pleasure is always face to face with pain. Life is meant to be unpredictably messy, exciting, and new, always new. Yin and Yang oscillate to provide the necessary tension to work out the raw material of our personal irritants. Like sand in an oyster, it is precisely our density and discomfort that we are meant to dance with; and sometimes the Divine Composer directs a slow dance with whatever internal pressures haunt us until we are able to become intimate with the origins of our dis-ease states and take them into a higher Mind. The soul gathers up these treasures during life and bestows them as gifts back to the Shen. The symptoms we might experience along the way can either be viewed as problems to eradicate, or invitations into the deeper waters where true healing happens. And the deeper we dare to go, the more we are able to integrate in and through our bodies. It is through the doorway of the most impenetrable anguish that the gates of Heaven open to liberate us from our density and propel us into the higher realms. Perhaps those of us with the most to overcome meet the alchemical requirements for the highest transformation, and also possess the most precious gifts to bestow in return.

If I have anything to contribute to the healing community it is this. We can't do it under the system we are presently under, and we can't do it alone.

We have everything we need to overcome every ailment and be restored to our eternal nature, which is always healed, always whole. It has been there within you all the time, awaiting your realization.

Let's quit our striving for some ideal state of healing and admit where we have lost our way. Almost everything in our pharmaceutical and nutraceutical apothecary is intended to provide symptom management at best. We've been fed a medical view that disease states are isolated diagnoses that stand on their own, and require their own medications. This is simply not true. The cluster of symptoms that are diagnosed as particular disease entities are only the result of an outmoded reductionist belief system. The only truth they have is that with which we endow them. There are really no such entities as cancer, diabetes, or depression. If we are not experiencing a state of health, it means we've veered off course, and unless we are blindly searching for external remedies, the answers are always found within. We are here to develop our souls and redeem Shen from Jing, or Heaven from Earth; although we seem to have it upside down. When we attempt only to preserve the body and its earthly existence, we compromise the gifts of the spirit, and give in to entropy.

In coming full circle, let's return to our initial discussion about death. When all attempts at healing have failed to keep us in this space-time dimension, let us remember that death is not a failure in healing. Indigenous cultures often view death as the ultimate healing, as we emerge from the contraction of this gravitational field to return to our cosmic origin. Perhaps saving lives is the greatest tragedy, and losing one's life is the greatest reward. What if we entered into the specter of death's realm and learned to befriend her? Characters like Odysseus, Psyche, Hercules, Orpheus, Aeneus, and Jesus all traveled to the realm of the dead, returning transformed. Rumi asked, *When was I ever made less by dying?* Some spiritual disciplines meditate on death to find the doorway to the inner sanctum where we are united with the Source and find what death cannot destroy. Even near-death experiences can awaken the recognition of one's true nature and invigorate one's sense of purpose.

When our corporeal soul ceases to exist, what remains? When the white hardness of our teeth and bones returns to the ground, and we enter the Mysterious Pass, we are left with Xuan, the mystery contained within the dark. The Mysterious Mother is dark within dark, where they cancel each other out. Beneath the darkness there is an unfathomable light, beyond our ideas of light and dark. It is the color of your head as far as your eyes are concerned; the luminosity that shines within the darkness and doesn't remove it. Perhaps *before* our teeth and bones return to the ground, we can let go of Metal's desire to control, and experience the deathless mystery now. Dying is a process of letting go of control; relinquishing the false identity, which is based on control, can begin at any time. Disentangling the ego structures allows us to return, "reborn" in the same body with a different outlook.

As the luck of the Tao would have it, as aging commences to deplete our stores of Jing, Qi, and Blood, while certain patterns of imbalance might be more likely to manifest, our means of holding our egocentric view of life together also unravels. For some, this causes tremendous suffering; yet the same process can also liberate. When we are connected to the Source, we do not need to steer our own agenda anymore and can return to the eternal longing of the soul which may have been neglected when we were desperately trying to keep it all together. When life presents those horrific opportunities (like illness) where all we're able to do is surrender to the inevitable, we have access to another source of power. The Great Mystery can kick in and work wonders if we are willing to relinquish our previous bearings.

The classical Taoist view of the birth/death spectrum of life allows us to peer into the ultimate mystery. It tells us that when we do succumb to bodily death, the Po will return to the ground, although fragments of their ghostly existence may continue to wander at the time and place of their death, especially when there are unreleased attachments or unfinished business. Quite paradoxically, it is through a process governed by the control cycle that we learn to surrender control; for the purpose of control is to keep things in place: homeo-*stasis*. The purpose of life itself might very well be its opposite. During fetal life, as Shen imparts our curriculum, the five elemental agents enter via the control cycle. As we birth into the death gate, the unraveling occurs in reverse order. The doorway to the unborn realm opens via inverse laws, but swings both ways.

As earthly thought structures relinquish control of Water, fear begins to dissipate. When Wood loses its control over Earth, the individual's appetite for earthly things is diminished. As Metal releases its hold on Wood, glitches in the memory may distort the previous Blood-based reality, giving us access to a wider lens that opens up the Hun to other dimensions. As Fire gives up its control over Metal, our wings unfurl and breathing patterns shift to a different, more irregular rhythm. And as Water lets go of Fire, our consciousness becomes aroused. During this last flicker, our cheeks may develop a rosy glow, and we become more spirited as Shen leaves its identification with the body. If you happen to have the honor of being present when someone is going through the relinquishment process, the entire atmosphere becomes charged with an effervescent aliveness. As the Po and Hun release their final embrace of this life, the animating force of the body atomizes into pure Spirit, and if you are rooted in Shen, you can sense there is nothing left but joy. The Shen, no longer energizing the Blood, vitalizes the field of Qi with the love that it is on return to its heavenly home.

While this process of release is occurring, and the transitioning where one is able to peer into distant lands and communicate with their inhabitants, some feel it is most important for the person to remain aware, with an unclouded Shen. If the patient is overly narcotized during this process, the Hun soul's ability to survey the entire landscape of its life to discover its true meaning may be sabotaged. The ethereal soul is here for a reason, which it must come to discover and report to the divine Emperor, especially at life's end. Narcotics damage the Liver and challenge one's sense of completion. If one's vision is clouded by opioids on the final journey of evocation, the process of relinquishing memories and attachments may be impeded; knowledge of one's very reason for being and their sense of purpose may become fractured and disoriented. The most important question, *What was my life about?*, never gets answered. This can cause Blood stasis in the Liver, traumatize the Pericardium, and interrupt the soul's process of letting go and moving on. As the Hun and Po souls exit the body, the Po may linger, while the Hun may be unable to integrate proper recall in life. This skews the Hun's vision, and without a proper life review, it is unable to get its bearings to move on. As the distorted Hun look for the light of Heaven or a subsequent incarnation to work out any unfinished business, the lack of integration may cause the soul to wander into its next life fragmented, confused as to its purpose, and potentially manifest conditions like autism or other mental disabilities.

While the Tao doesn't make mistakes, humans do tend to lose harmony with nature. It appears we are in the midst of a very challenging collective lesson—no matter how smart we think we've become, we can't improve on the great nature of reality. Our human vision is too limited. Science is thus further limited. And its child, conventional medicine, is the most narrow of focus. Perhaps our interference with the process of life and death is responsible for the rise in many of the disorders we are experiencing today. Yet the truth of the Tao lives in the Heart of every cell and can be resurrected at any time.

We've been living upside down. White are the mountain peaks, sterilized cleanliness, and the bones of death. Black is the unknown but always fertile vale where the mysterious origin resides. Let's stop our striving to control, to medicate life, and return to the Valley, where the entire universe can enter and steer us back to truth. The Tao beckons us to recognize that *the Valley Spirit never dies*. While it might not be a popular belief that the macrocosm and the microcosm are one, to experience this reality is the most powerful recognition in life. We all intuit or at least have an inkling that there is an indwelling power, that we are miraculous expressions of the Tao, and all true healing comes from within. But we first have to cultivate this power and bring it into expression. The Tao won't interfere with our limiting beliefs or the actions which stem from them. It's our job to develop the courage of Heart to reside in the mystery and learn to utilize the Tao's tools. Many have experienced the most radical healing power when they dared to refuse to be medicated—surrendering to something outside the expected, predictable man-made offerings. Only then were they receptive to the touch of the Spirit, for the Tao knows how to reach in and heal what needs to be healed.

We become sick and ail because we love what deceives us. In this state of mind, we value that which we know, and bow to homeostasis as the highest model. In the mind of Newtonian cause and effect, the conventional scientific method based on separation and division still rules. It believes we ail because something has gone wrong, that life has let us down, but medicine can fix the broken machines we have become. Real cures don't fix, but heal those who are willing to be healed. When its aim is to cleanse the orifices and open the portals, we can become receptive on every level to a new way of being, based on the quantum view that we are One, integral to the family of the ten thousand things, and the power of healing is always at hand. What are you loyal to—entropy, which is governed by fear of physical demise, or alchemy, where the power of transformation rules? This is a time of hope, and we in the field of Asian medicine are poised to be part of a desperately needed solution. The Valley Spirit is eternal, always at hand, and will never run dry. As we heal one person at a time, the whole world changes.

References

Abramson, J. (2013) Should people at low risk of cardiovascular disease take a statin? *British Medical Journal*, 347: f6123. doi: https://doi.org/10.1136/bmj.f6123.

Baguley, B.C. (2002) A Brief History of Cancer Chemotherapy. http://marc.barritault.bio.free.fr/Anticancer%20Drug%20Development/Chapter01.pdf.

Bar-Shalom, A. & Cook-Deegan, R. (2002) Patents and innovation in cancer therapeutics: Lessons from CellPro. *Milbank Quarterly*, 80(4): 637–676. doi: 10.1111/1468-0009.00027.

Blevins Primeau, A.S. (2023) Survey: Most Cancer Patients Use Complementary or Alternative Medicine. Cancer Therapy Advisor. www.cancertherapyadvisor.com/home/cancer-topics/general-oncology/survey-most-cancer-patients-use-complementary-or-alternative-medicine.

BMJ (2019) *Appropriateness of outpatient antibiotic prescribing among privately insured US patients: ICD-10-CM based cross sectional study*. https://doi.org/10.1136/bmj.k5092

Briggs, A.D.M., Mizdrak, A., & Scarborough, P. (2013) A statin a day keeps the doctor away: Comparative proverb assessment modelling study. *British Medical Journal*, 347: f7267. doi: https://doi.org/10.1136/bmj.f7267.

Can we make cancer cells normal again? (2017) Columbia University Irving Medical Center. www.cuimc.columbia.edu/news/can-we-make-cancer-cells-normal-again.

DeVita, Jr., V.T. & Chu, E. (2008) A history of cancer chemotherapy. *Cancer Research*, 68(21): 8643–8653. http://cancerres.aacrjournals.org/content/68/21/8643.full.pdf.

Dorr, R.T. & Paxinos, J. (1978) The current status of laetrile. *Annals of Internal Medicine*, 89(3): 389–397.

DuBroff, R., Malhotra, A., & de Lorgeril, M. (2021) Hit or miss: The new cholesterol targets. *BMJ Evidence-Based Medicine*, 26(6): 271–278. doi: 10.1136/bmjebm-2020-111413.

Dunleavy, K. (2022) The Top 20 drugs by worldwide sales in 2021. *Fierce Pharma*. www.fiercepharma.com/special-reports/top-20-drugs-worldwide-sales-2021

Finucane, M.M., Stevens, G.A., Cowan, M.J. *et al.* (2011) National, regional, and global trends in body-mass index since 1980: Systematic analysis of health examination surveys and epidemiological studies with 960 country-years and 9.1 million participants. *The Lancet*, 377(9765): 557–567.

Gurgula, O. (2020) Strategic patenting by pharmaceutical companies—Should competition law intervene? *International Review of Intellectual Property and Competition Law*, 51(9): 1062–1085. doi: 10.1007/s40319-020-00985-0.

Hay, J.H. (1931) A British Medical Association Lecture on The Significance of a Raised Blood Pressure. *British Medical Journal*, 2(3679): 43–47. doi: 10.1136/bmj.2.3679.43.

How John D. Rockefeller influenced modern medicine (n.d.) www.potency710.com/how-john-d-rockefeller-influenced-modern-medicine.

How Rockefeller created the business of Western medicine (2019) Meridian Health Clinic. https://meridianhealthclinic.com/how-rockefeller-created-the-business-of-western-medicine.

JEC (n.d.) *The Economic Toll of the Opioid Crisis Reached Nearly $1.5 Trillion in 2020*. www.jec.senate.gov/public/_cache/files/67bced7f-4232-40ea-9263-f033d280c567/jec-cost-of-opioids-issue-brief.pdf

Karlis, N. (2019) Why Dr. Zach Bush believes herbicides could end life on Earth. Salon. Available at: www.salon.com/2019/10/14/why-dr-zach-bush-believes-herbicides-could-end-life-on-earth.

Lewis, R. (2022) *Spirit of the Blood*. London: Singing Dragon.

Malhotra, A. (2013) Saturated fat is not the major issue. *British Medical Journal*, 347: f6340. doi: https://doi.org/10.1136/bmj.f6340.

Mandal, A. (2023) History of Chemotherapy. News Medical. www.news-medical.net/health/History-of-Chemotherapy.aspx.

Maté, G. (2011) When the Body Says No. *Trade Paper Press*, January 1.

Meyers, D.E. *et al.* (2021) Trends in drug revenue among major pharmaceutical companies: A 2010-2019 cohort study. *American Cancer Society Journals*. https://doi.org/10.1002/cncr.33934.

Moss, R.W. (1996) Laetrile at Sloan-Kettering: A Case Study. In *The Cancer Industry: The Classic Expose on the Cancer Establishment* (pp.153–186). Brooklyn, NY: First Equinox Press.

Rasmussen, N. (2008) America's first amphetamine epidemic 1929-1971. *American Journal of Public Health*, 98(6): 974–985. doi: 10.2105/AJPH.2007.110593.

Rasmussen, N. (2011) Medical science and the military: The Allies' use of amphetamine during World War II. *Journal of Interdisciplinary History*, 42(2): 205–233. doi: 10.1162/jinh_a_00212.

Rauws, A.G., Olling, M., & Timmerman, A. (1982) The pharmacokinetics of prunasin, a metabolite of amygdalin. *Journal of Clinical Toxicology*, 19(8): 851–856.

Rosse de Souza, V., Concentino Menezes Brum, M., dos Santos Guimarães, I. *et al.* (2019) Amazon fruits inhibit growth and promote pro-apoptotic effects on human ovarian carcinoma cell lines. *Biomolecules*, 9(11): 707. doi: 10.3390/biom9110707.

Royal Pharmaceutical Society (2022) *The Pharmaceutical Journal*, July, 309(7963).

Rubik, B., Muehsam, D., Hammerschlag, R., & Jain, S. (2015) Biofield science and healing: History, terminology, and concepts. *Global Advances in Integrative Medicine and Health*, 4(Suppl): 8–14. doi: 10.7453/gahmj.2015.038.suppl.

Ruochen Dong, B.S., Ping Chen, M.S., & Qi Chen, PhD (2018) Extract of the medicinal plant pao pereira inhibits pancreatic cancer stem-like cell in vitro and in vivo. *Integrative Cancer Therapies*, 17(4): 1204–1215. doi: 10.1177/1534735418786027.

Sarno, J. (1999) *Mind Over Back Pain*. New York, NY: Berkley Press.

Shir Itai, Y., Oren Barboy, O., Salomon, R. *et al.* (2024) Bispecific dendritic-T cell engager potentiates anti-tumor immunity. *Cell*, 187(2): 375–389.

Stephenson, C. (2017) *The Acupuncturist's Guide to Conventional Medicine*, Appendix 2. London: Singing Dragon.

Valk, S., Bernhardt, B.C., Trautwein, F.-M. *et al.* (2017) Structural plasticity of the social brain: Differential change after socio-affective and cognitive mental training. *Science Advances*, 3(10). doi: 10.1126/sciadv.1700489.

Zwawiak, J. & Zaprutko, L. (2014) A brief history of taxol. *Journal of Medical Science*, 83(1): 47–52. doi: https://doi.org/10.20883/medical.e43.

Bibliography

Chandler, R.F., Anderson, L.A., & Phillipson, J.D. (1984) Laetrile in perspective. *Canadian Pharmacists Journal*, 117(11): 517–520.

Curt, G.A. (1990) Unsound methods of cancer treatment. *Principles of Practical Oncology Updates*, 4(12): 1–10.

Ellison, N.M., Byar, D.P., & Newell, G.R. (1978) Special report on Laetrile: The NCI Laetrile Review. Results of the National Cancer Institute's retrospective Laetrile analysis. *New England Journal of Medicine*, 299(10): 549–552.

Herbert, V. (1979) Laetrile: The cult of cyanide. Promoting poison for profit. *American Journal of Clinical Nutrition*, 32(5): 1121–1158.

Howard-Ruben, J. & Miller, N.J. (1984) Unproven methods of cancer management. Part II: Current trends and implications for patient care. *Oncology Nursing Forum*, 11(1): 67–73.

Lerner, I.J. (1981) Laetrile: A lesson in cancer quackery. *CA: A Cancer Journal for Clinicians*, 31(2): 91–95.

Lewis, J.P. (1977) Laetrile. *West Journal of Medicine*, 127(1): 55–62.

Moertel, C.G., Fleming, T.R., Rubin, J. *et al.* (1982) A clinical trial of amygdalin (Laetrile) in the treatment of human cancer. *New England Journal of Medicine*, 306(4): 201–206.

Moss, R.W. (1996) The Laetrile Controversy. In *The Cancer Industry: The Classic Expose on the Cancer Establishment* (pp.131–152). Brooklyn, NY: First Equinox Press.

Newmark, J., Brady, R.O., Grimley, P.M. *et al.* (1981) Amygdalin (Laetrile) and prunasin beta-glucosidases: Distribution in germ-free rat and in human tumor tissue. *Proceedings of the National Academy of Sciences of the USA*, 78(10): 6513–6516.

Rosen, G.M. & Shorr, R.I. (1979) Laetrile: End play around the FDA. A review of legal developments. *Annals of Internal Medicine*, 90(3): 418–423.

Ross, W.E. (1985) Unconventional cancer therapy. *Comprehensive Therapy*, 11(9): 37–43.

Unproven methods of cancer management. Laetrile. (1972) *CA: A Cancer Journal for Clinicians*, 22(4): 245–250.

Viehoever, A. & Mack, H. (1935) Bio-chemistry of amygdalin (bitter, cyanogenetic principle from bitter almonds). *American Journal of Pharmaceutical Education*, 107 (Oct): 397–450.